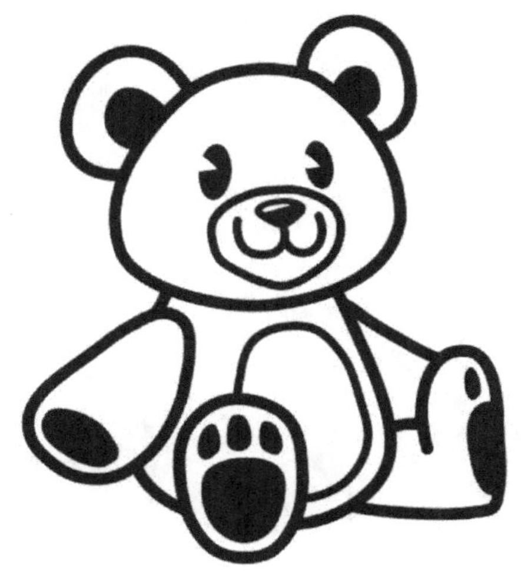

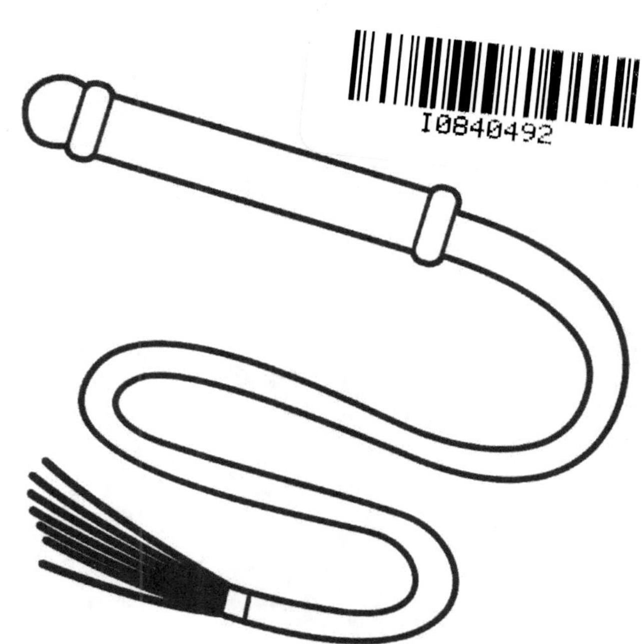

This Book Belongs To

____

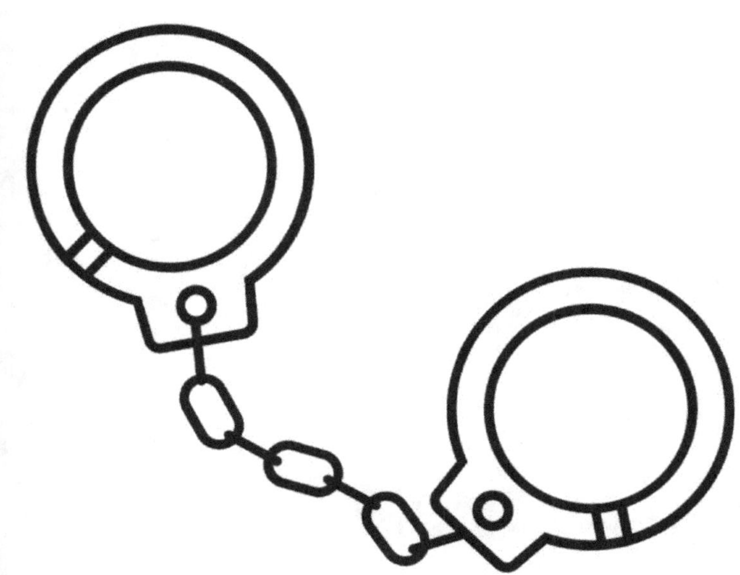

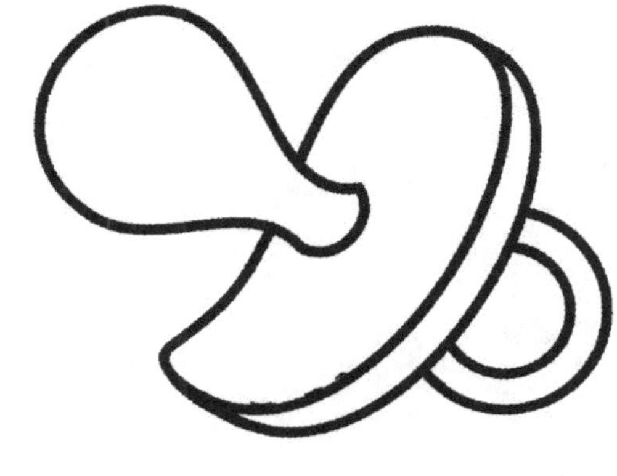

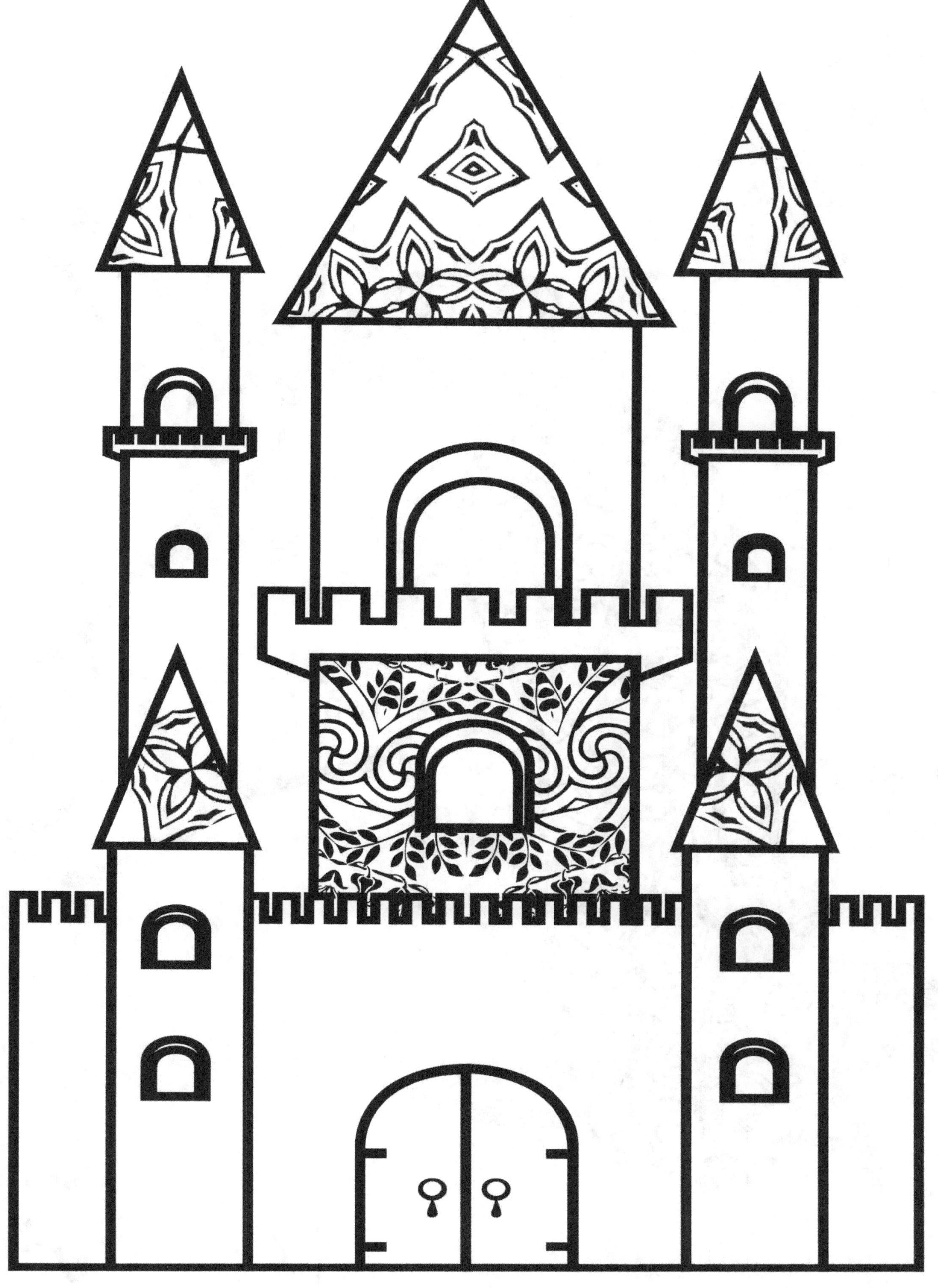

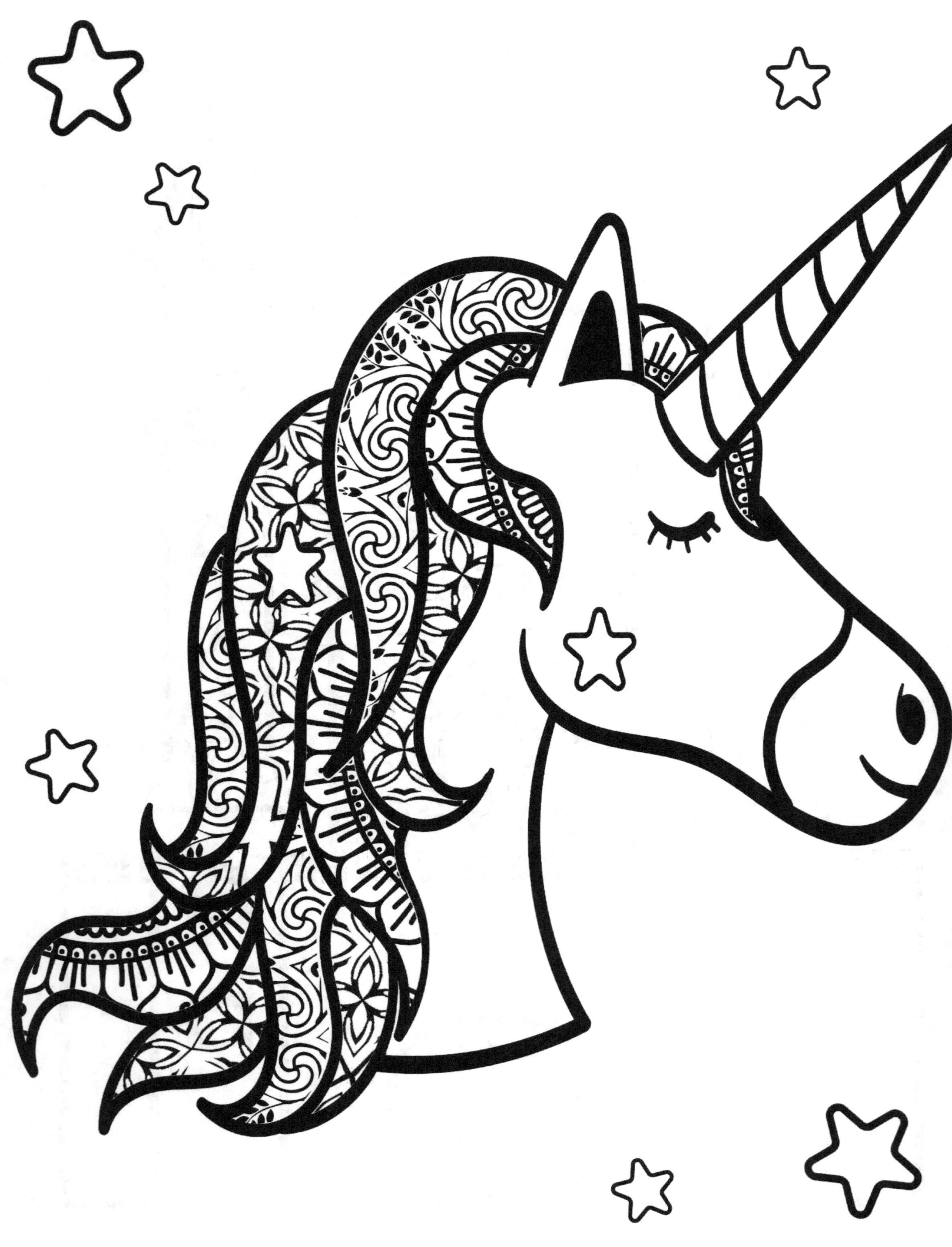

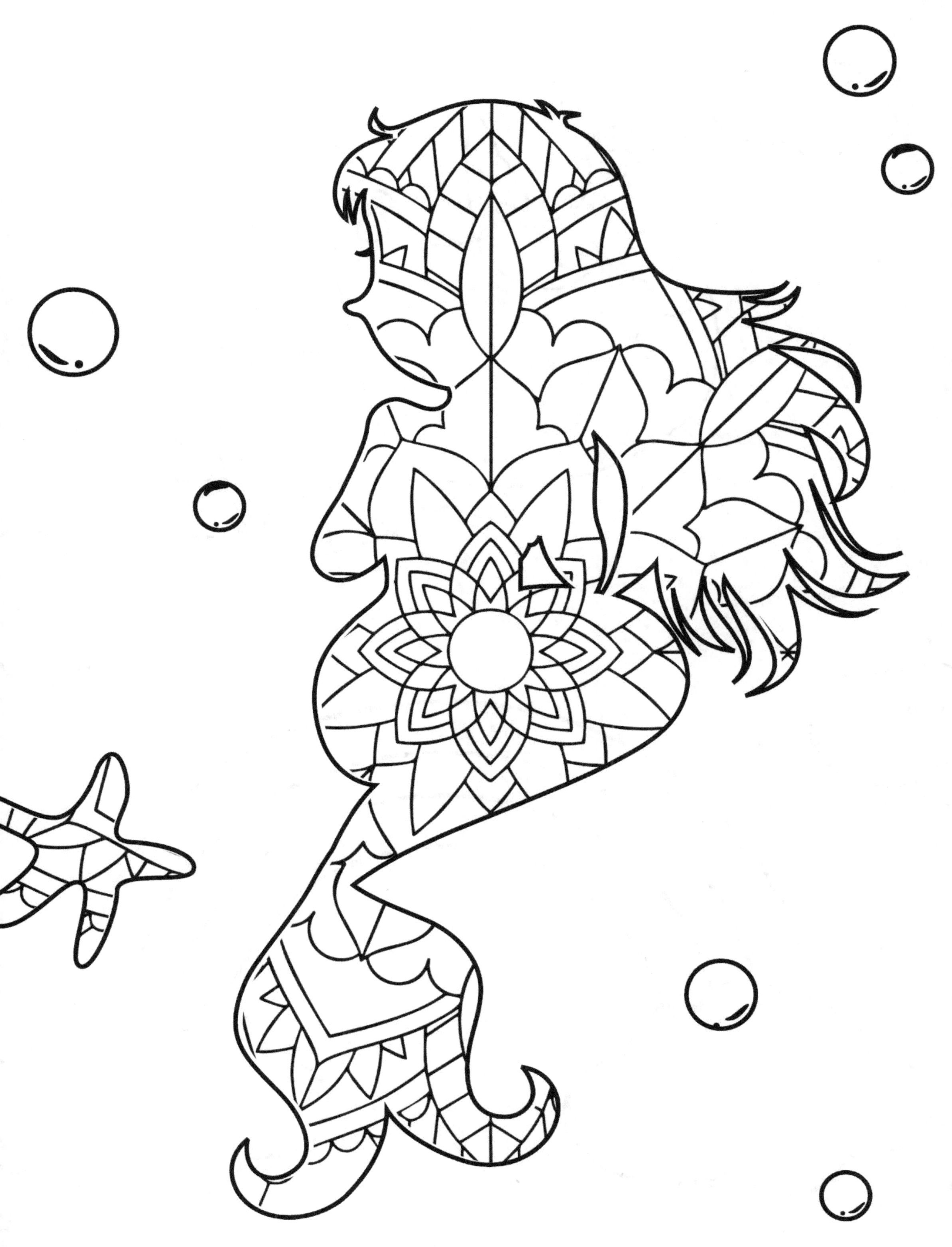

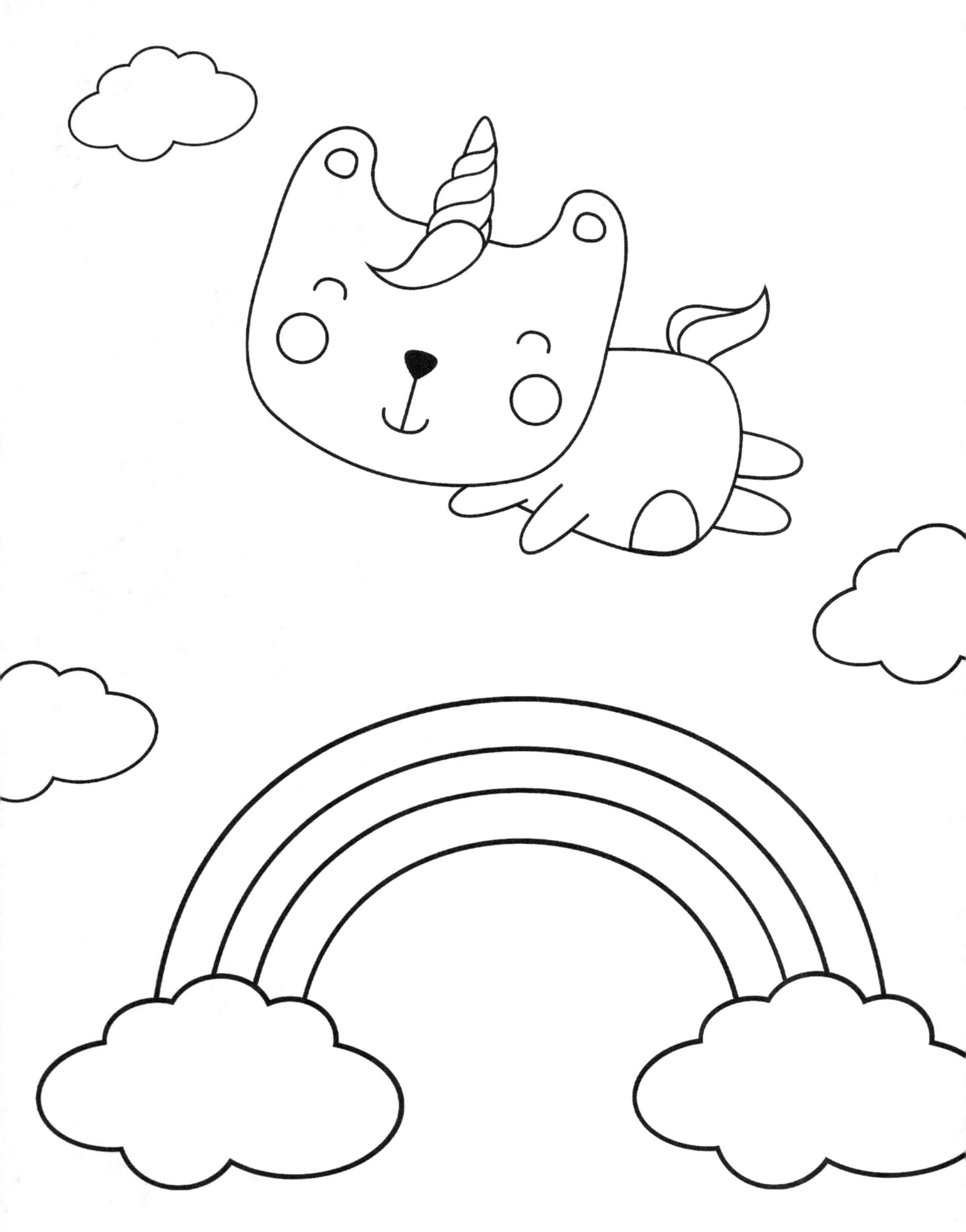

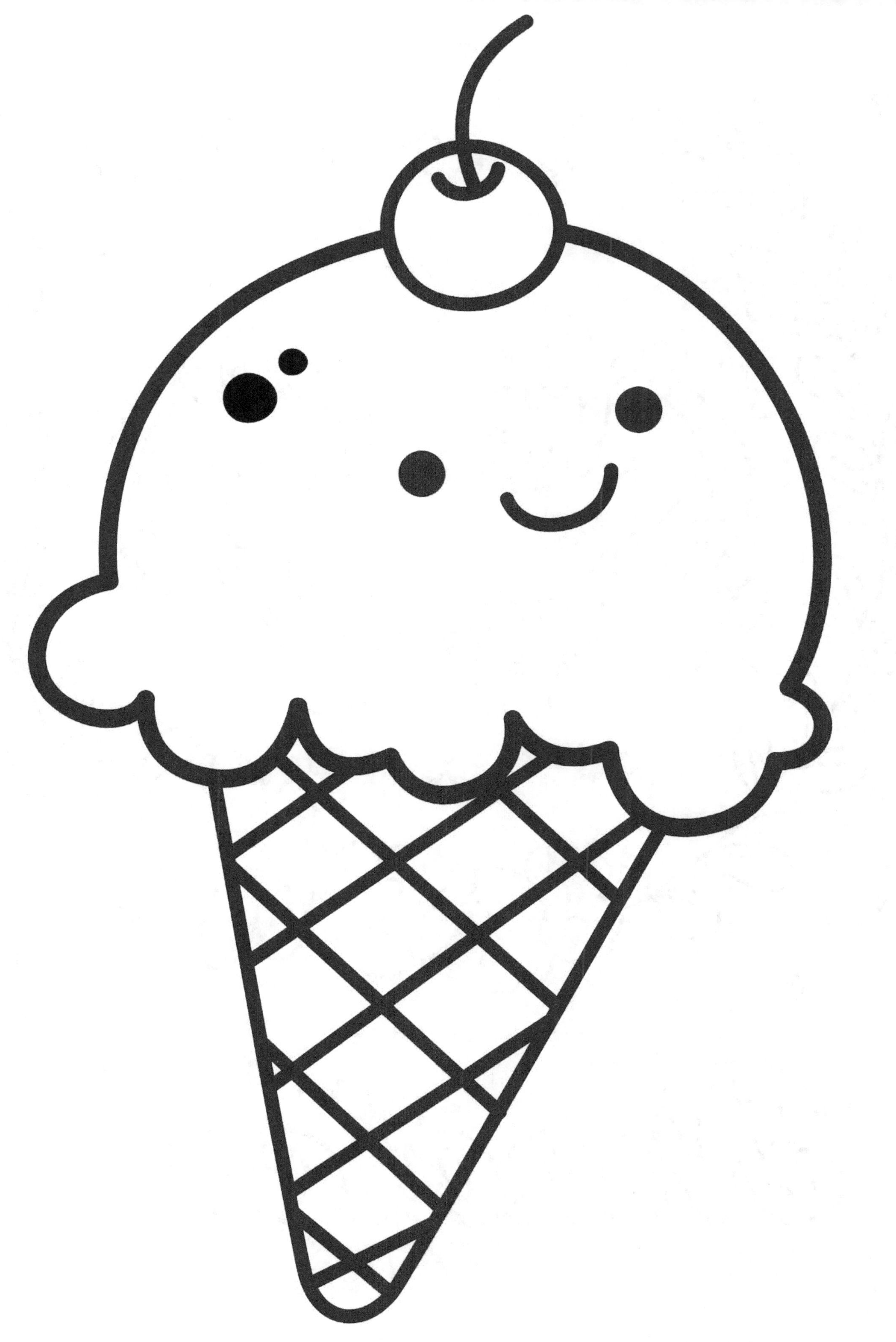

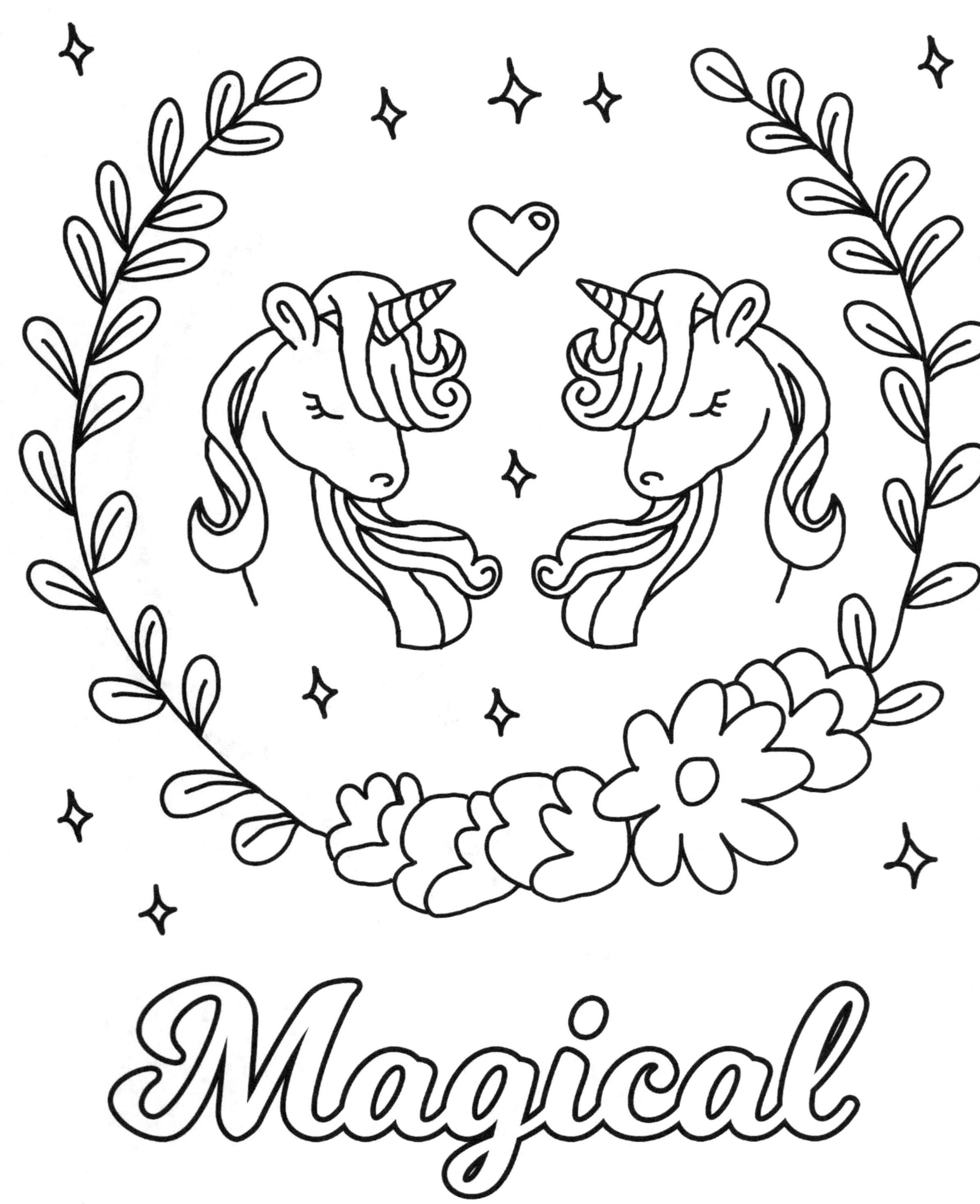

Magical

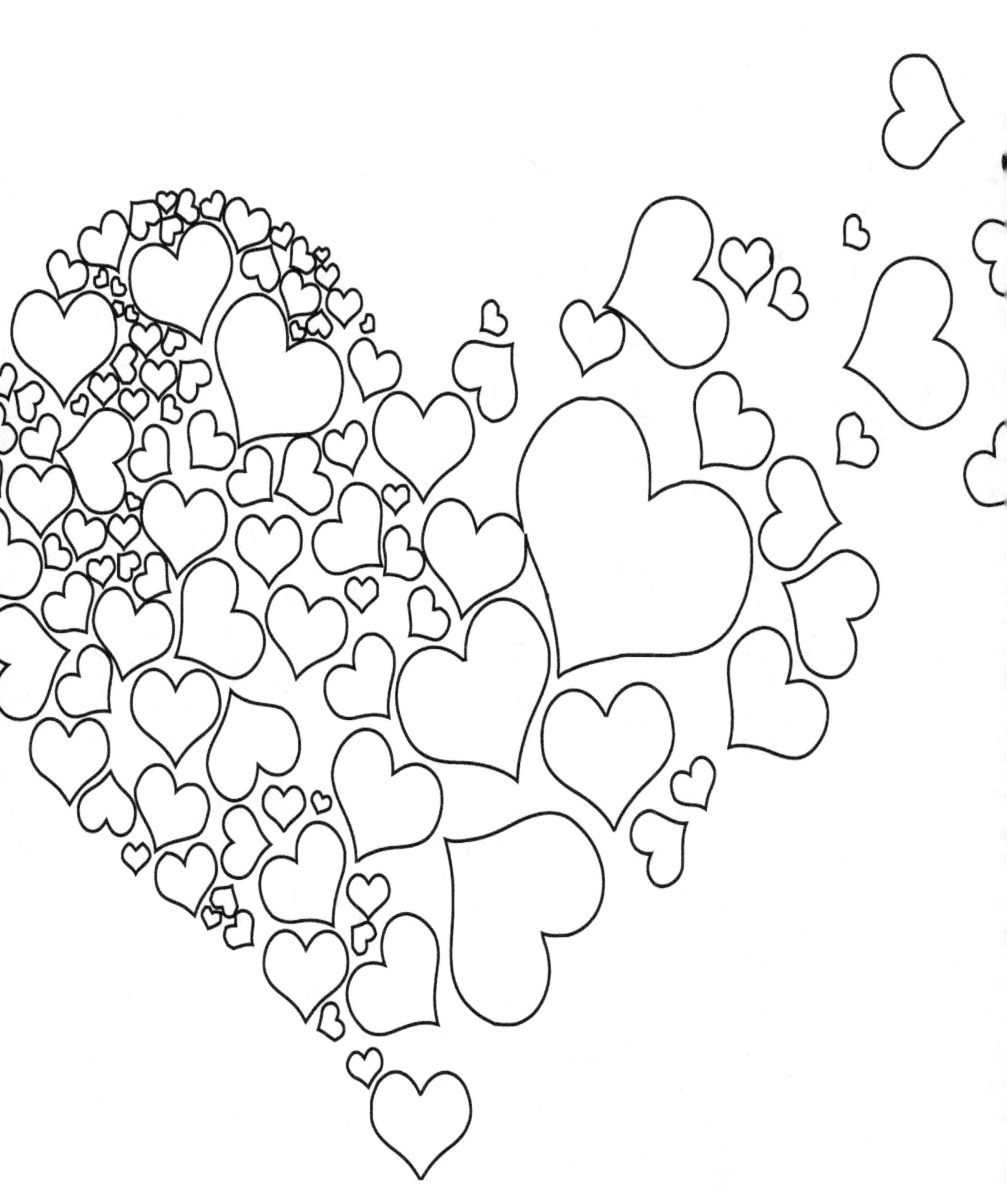

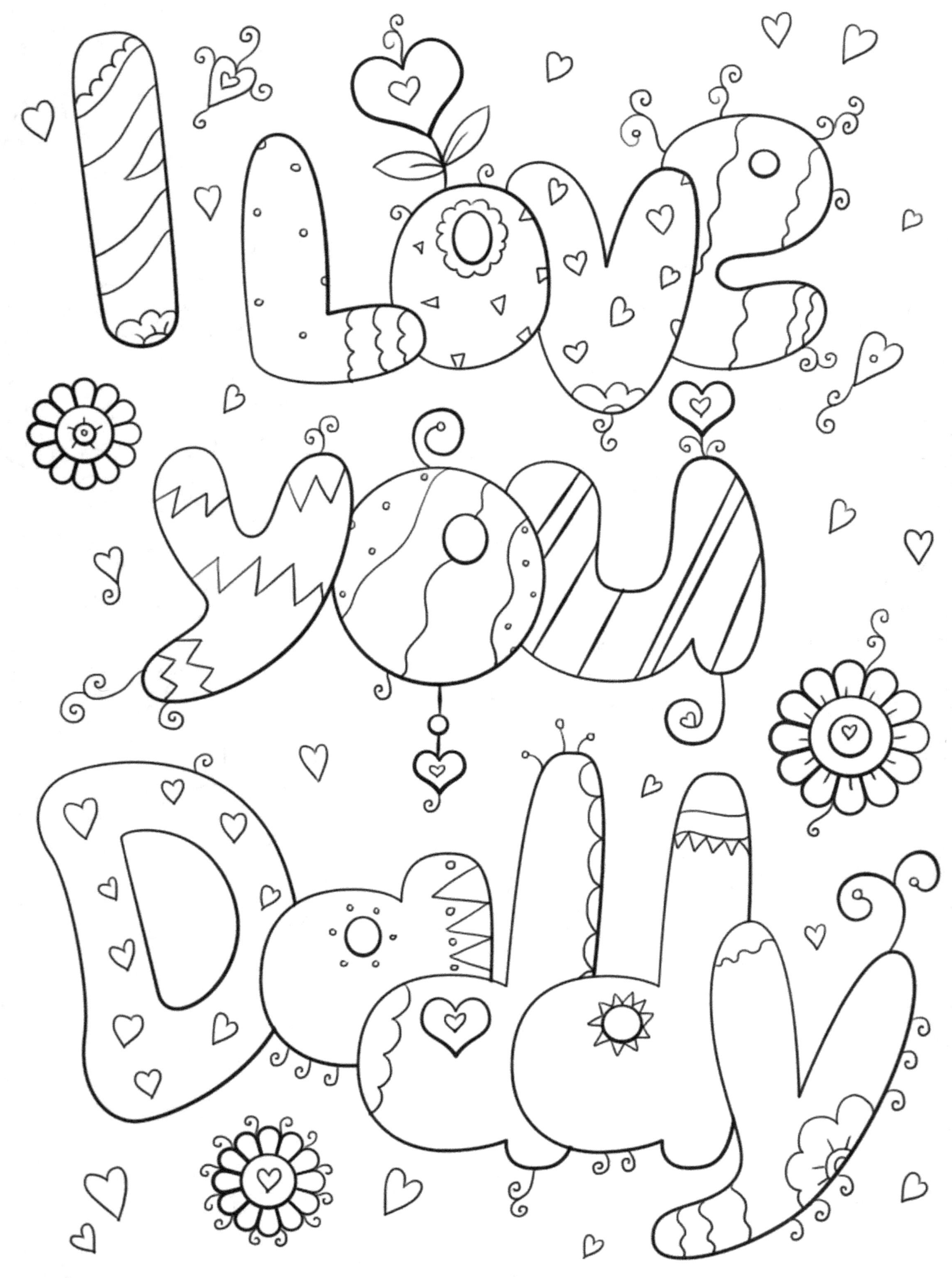

I Love you
Daddy

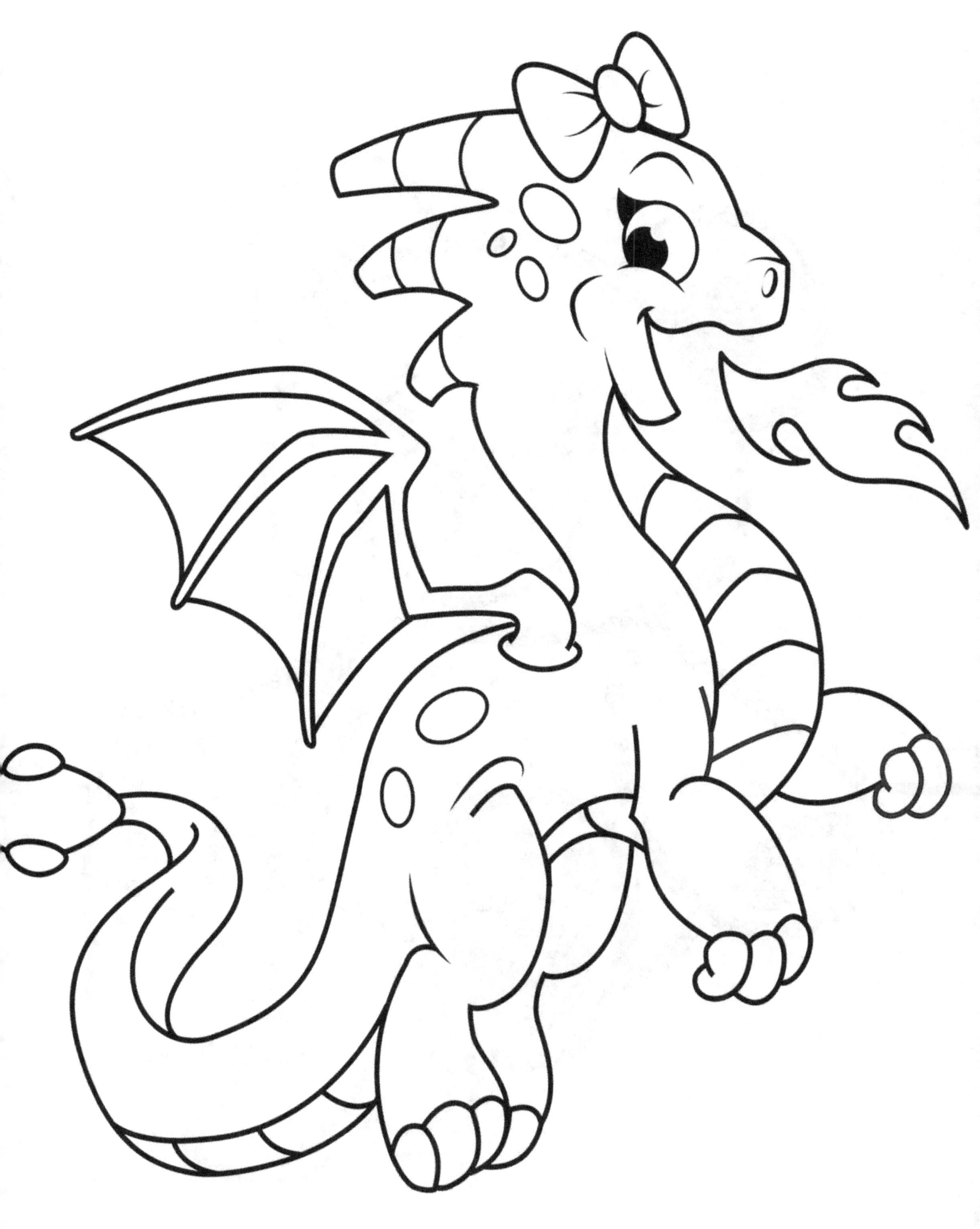

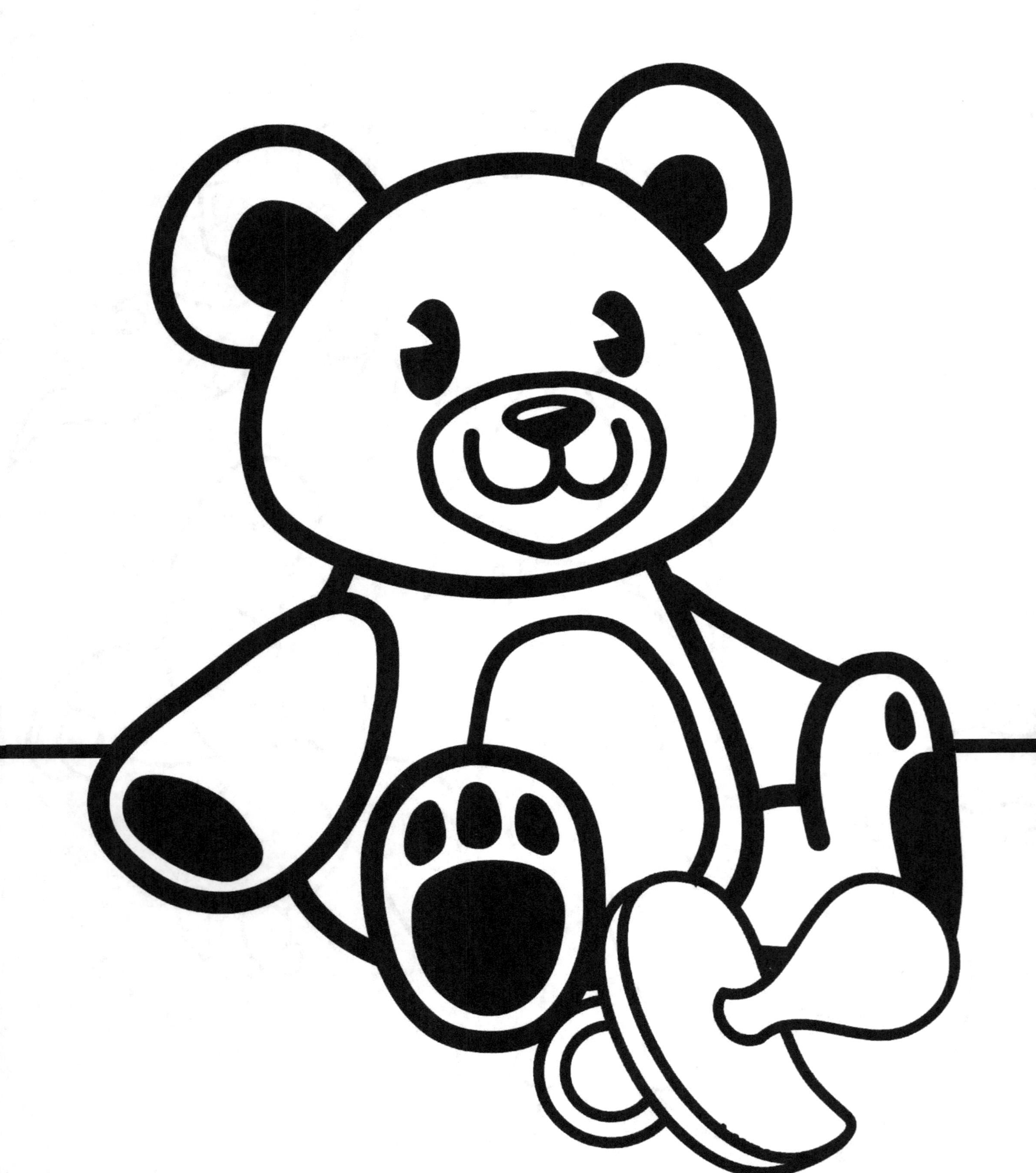

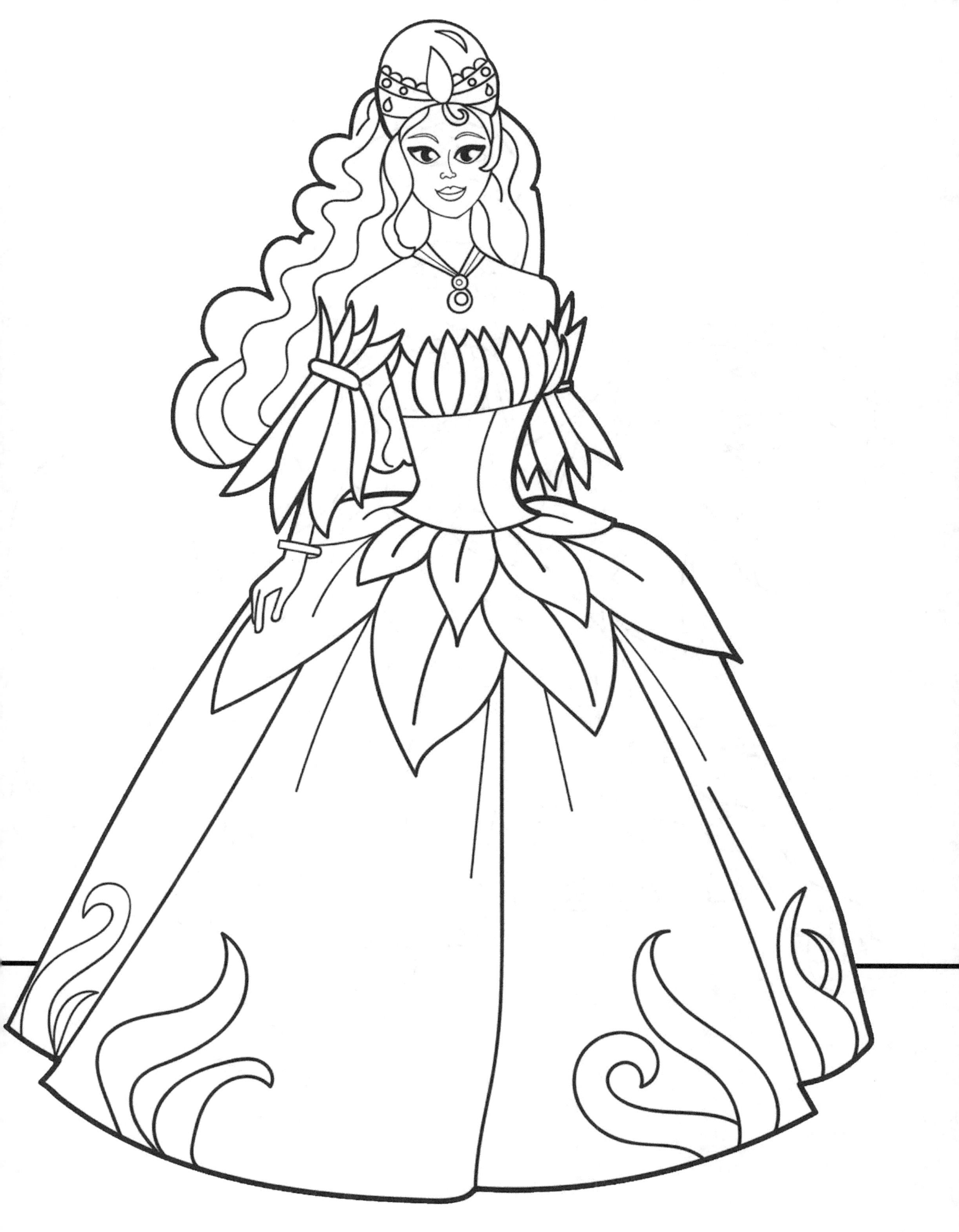

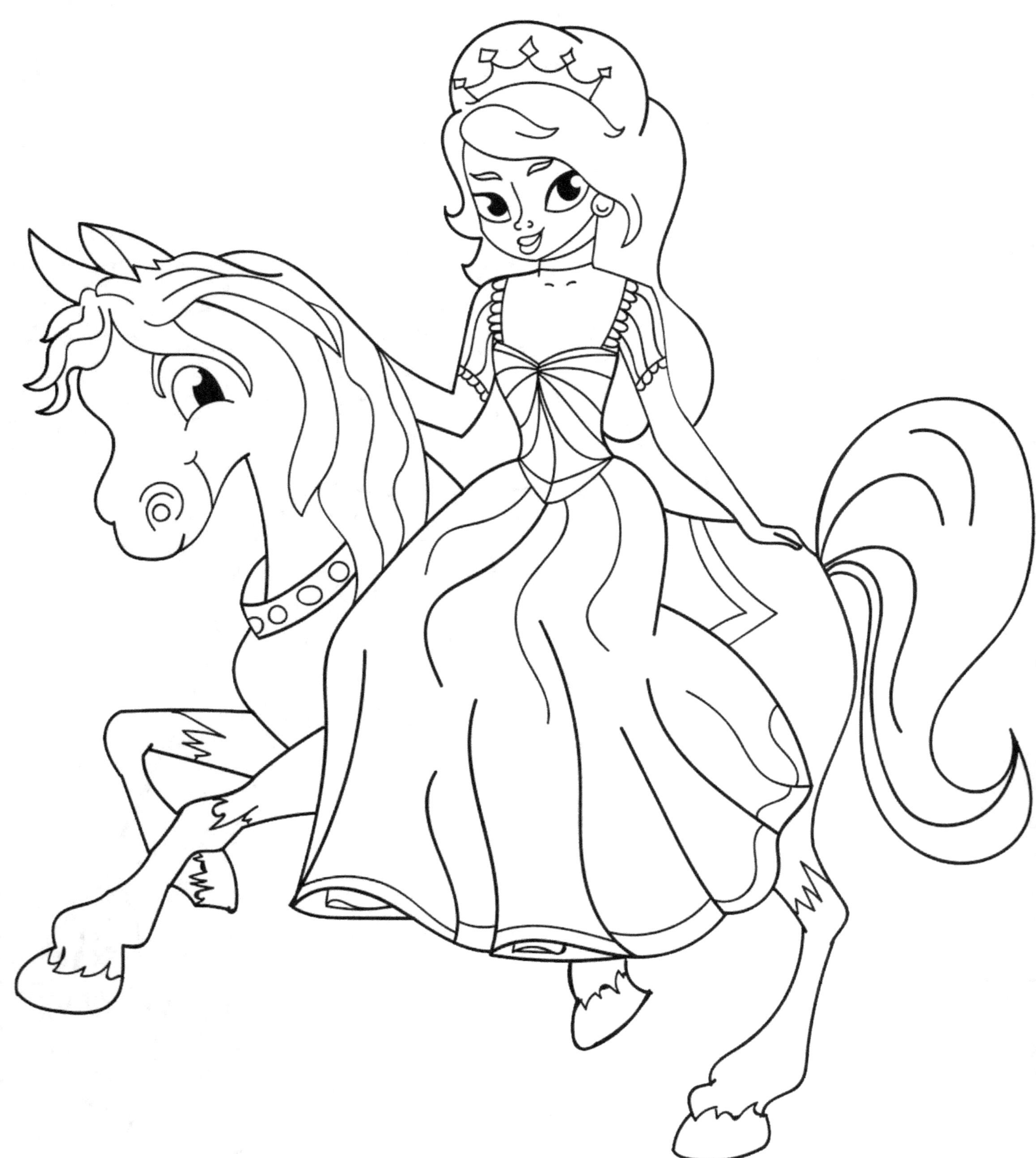

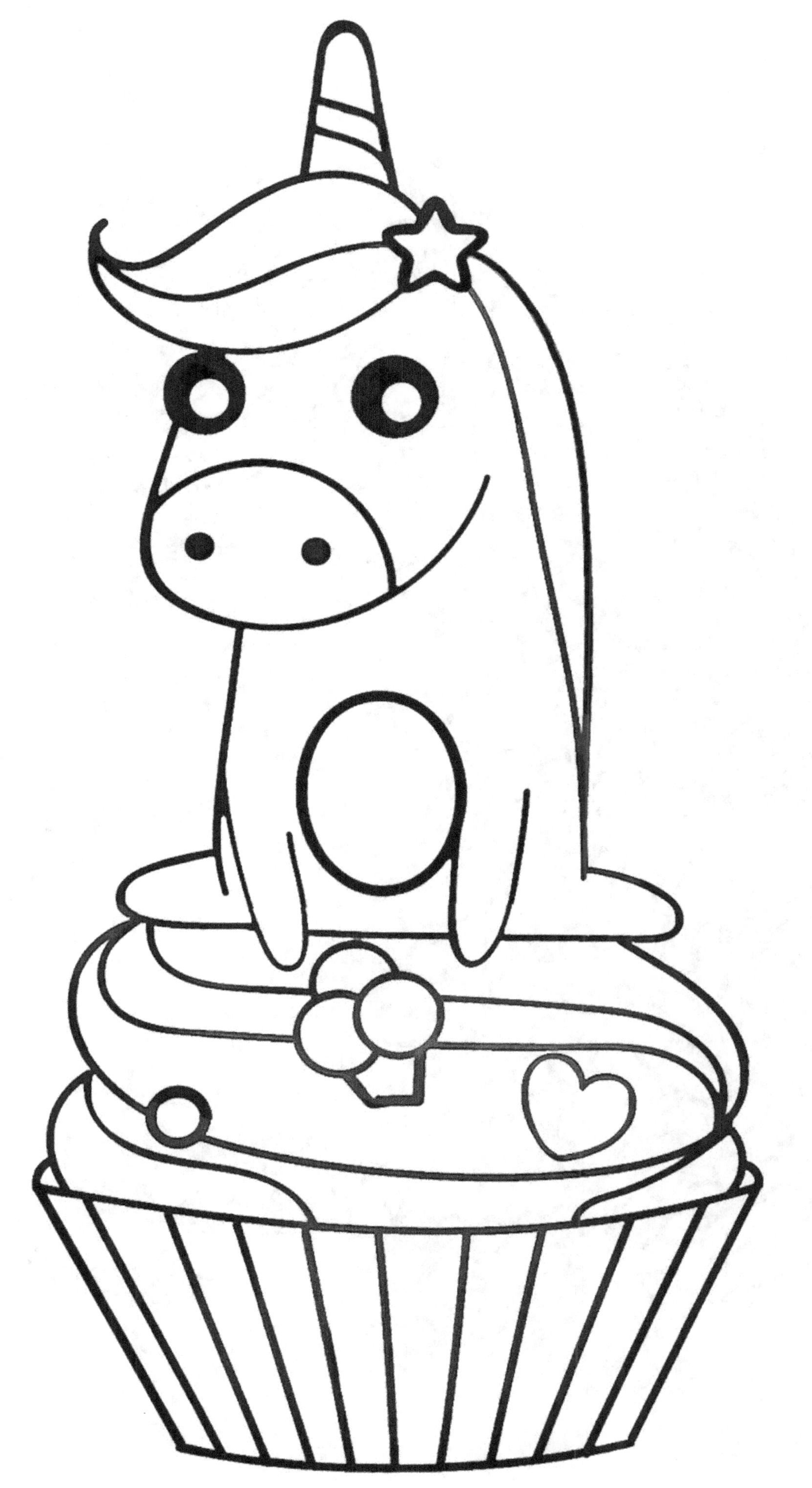

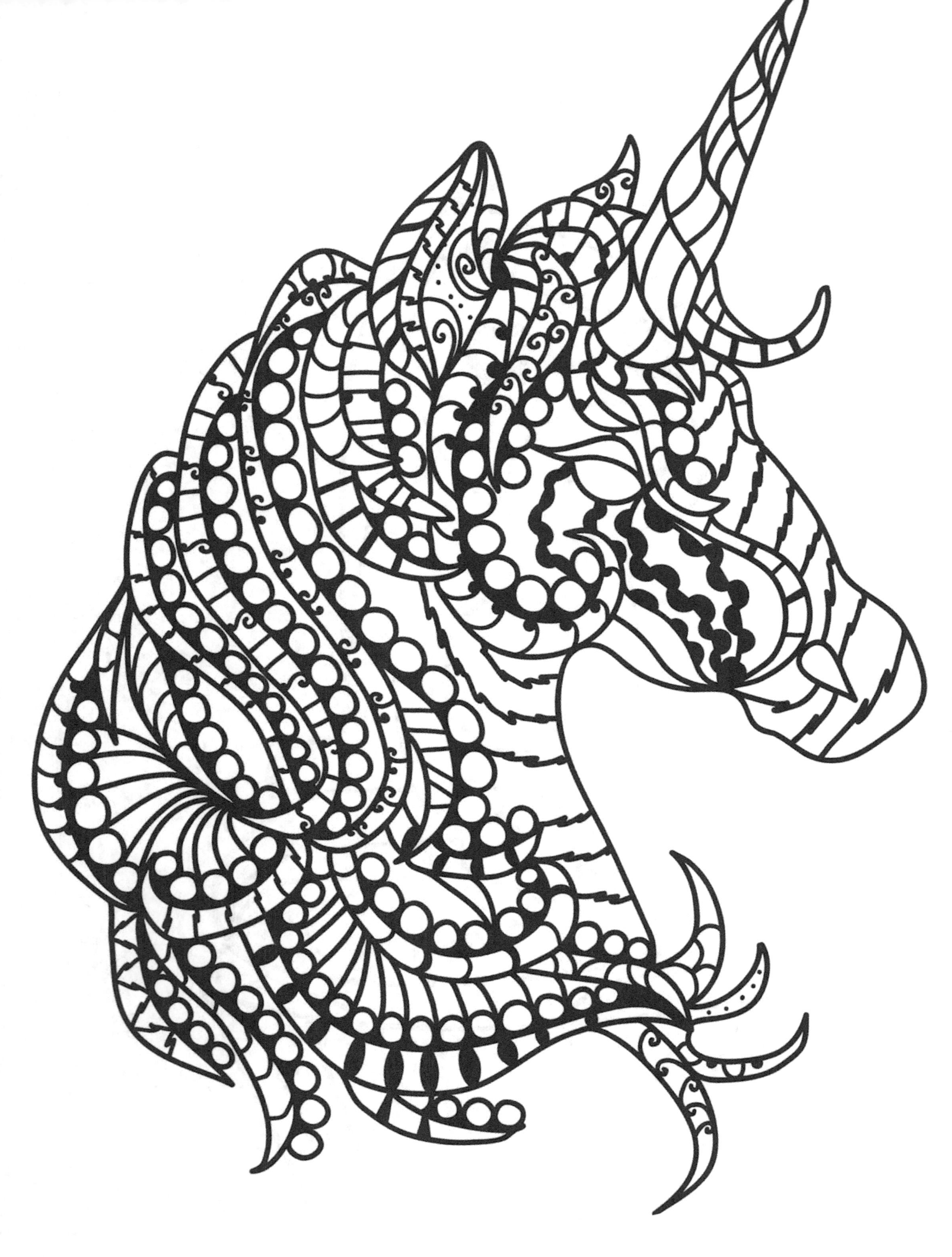

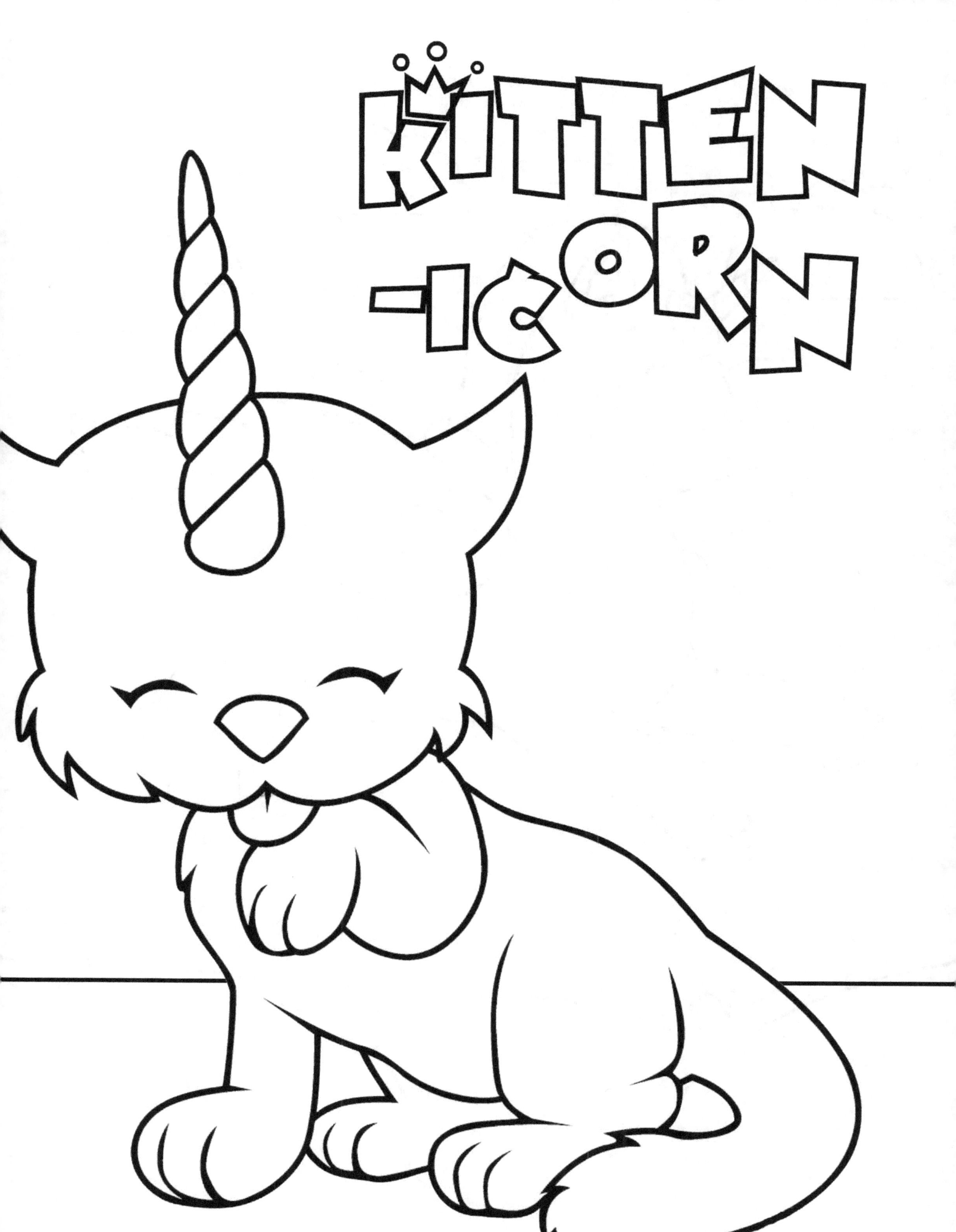

KITTEN
-ICORN

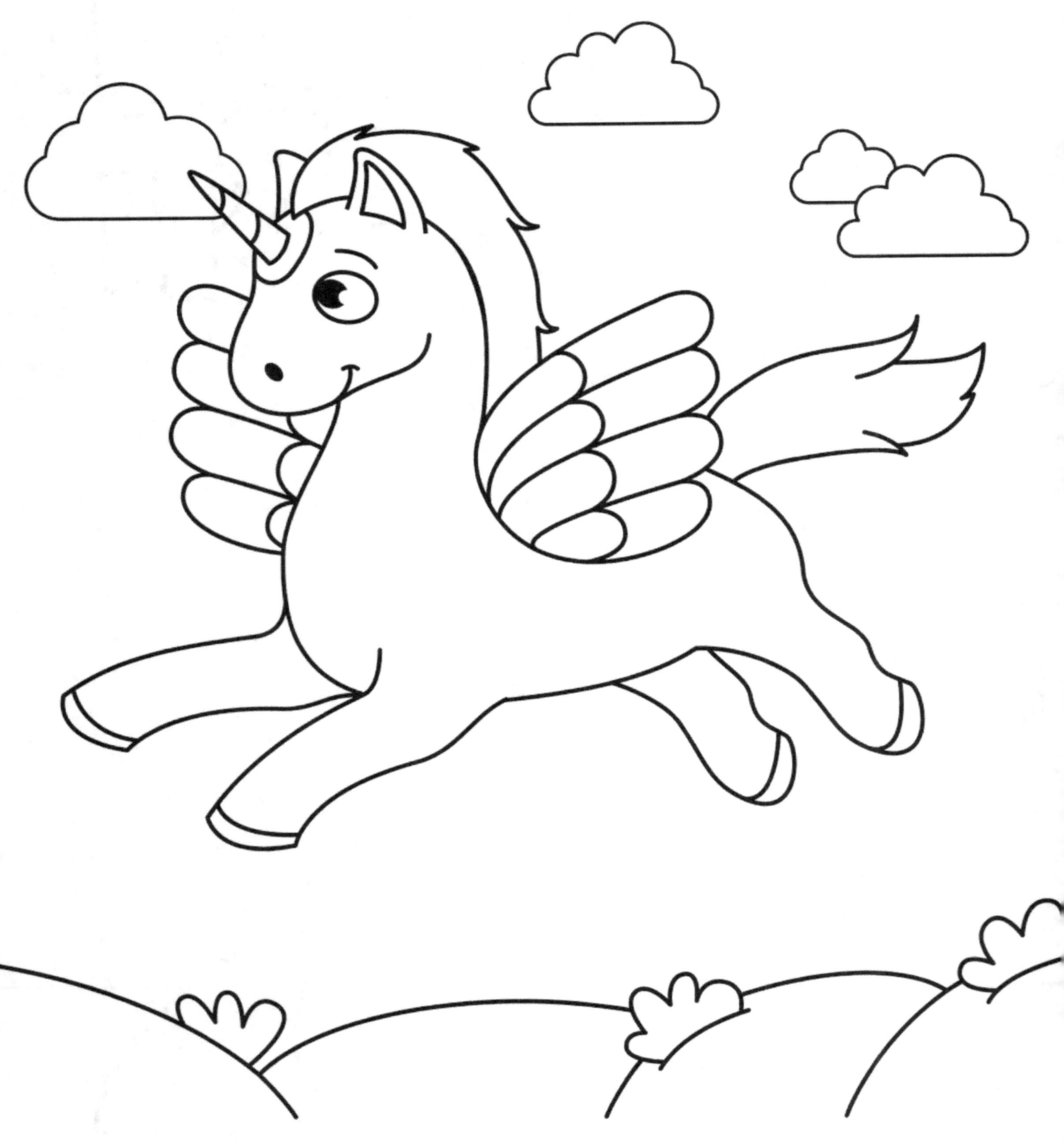

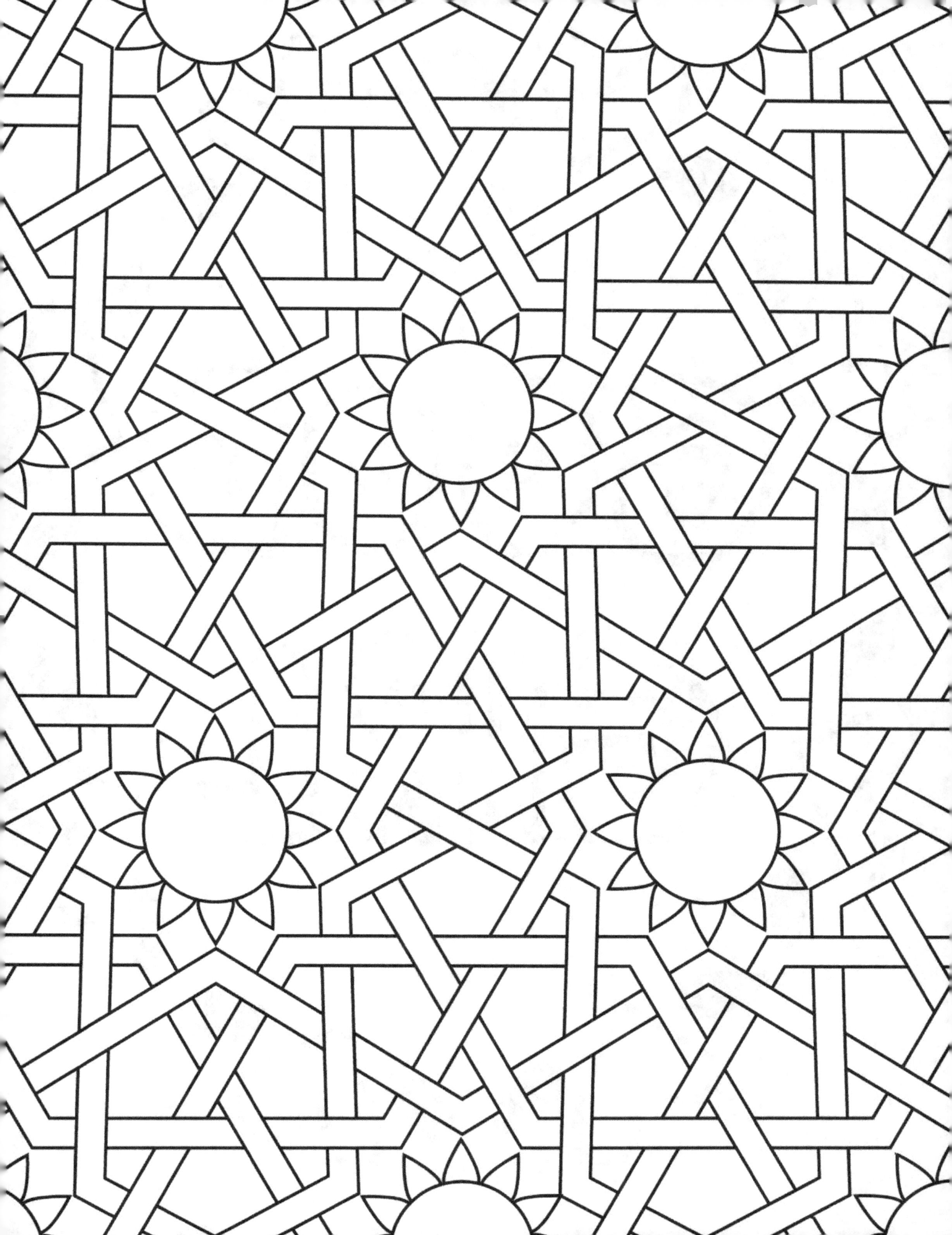

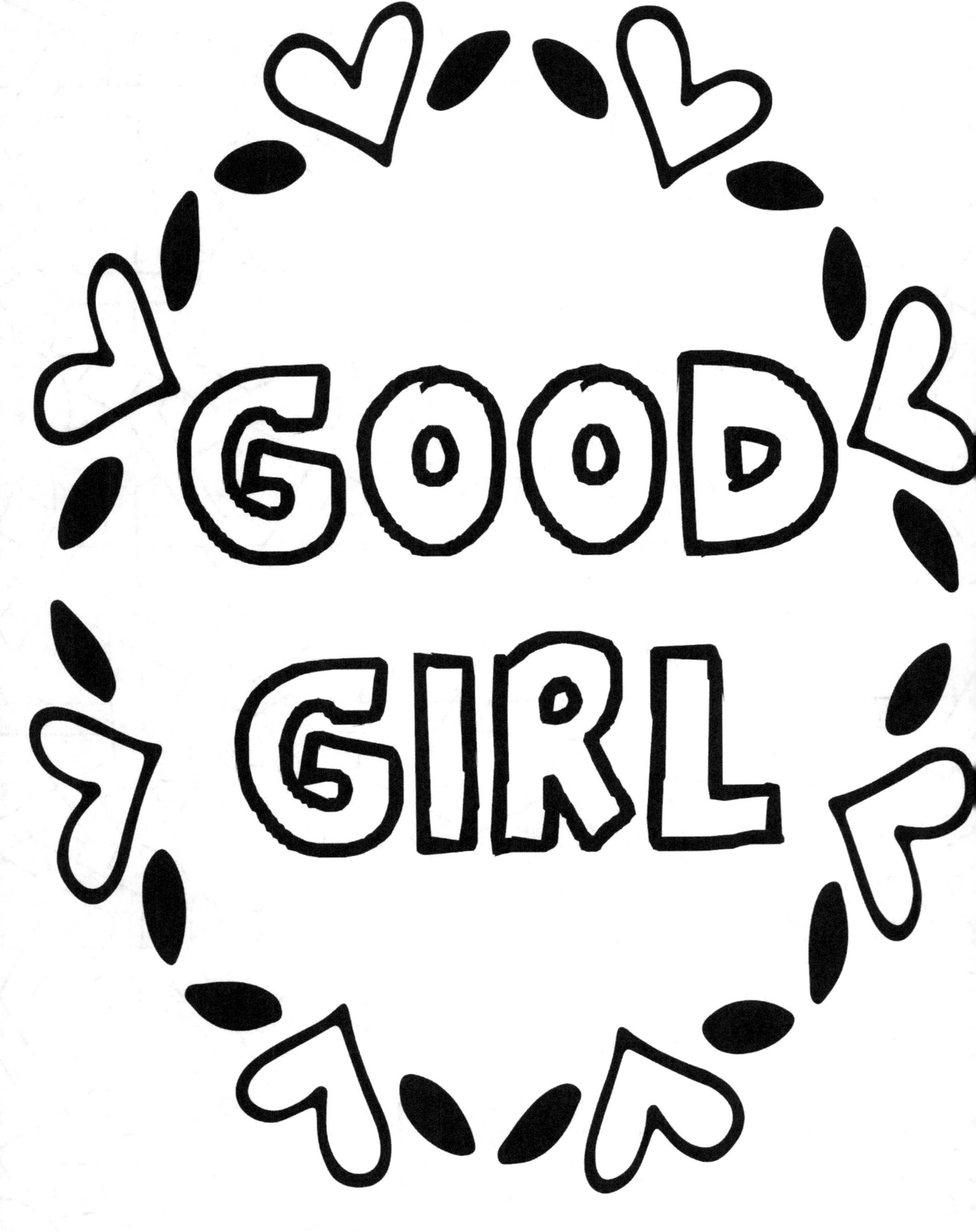

GOOD
GIRL

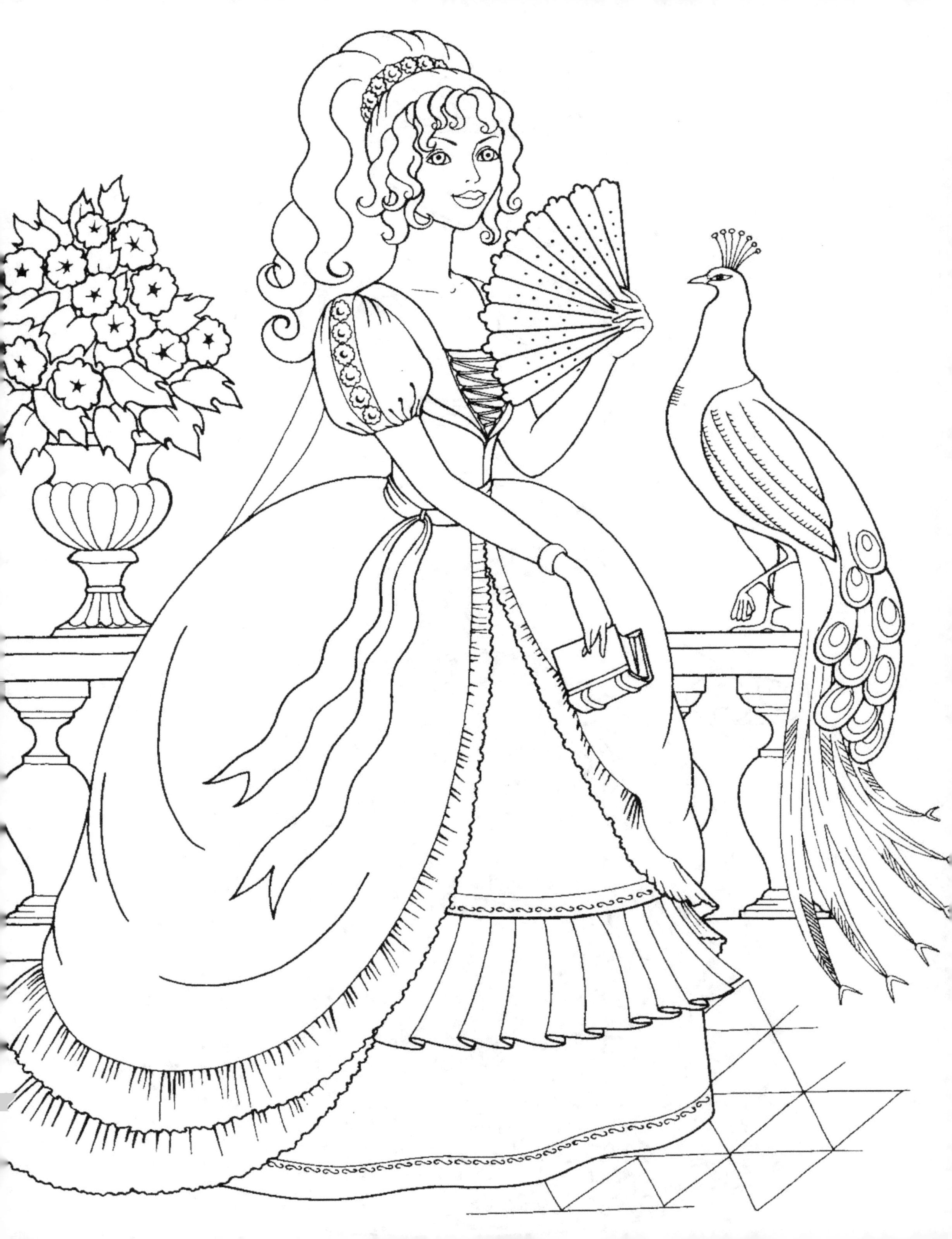

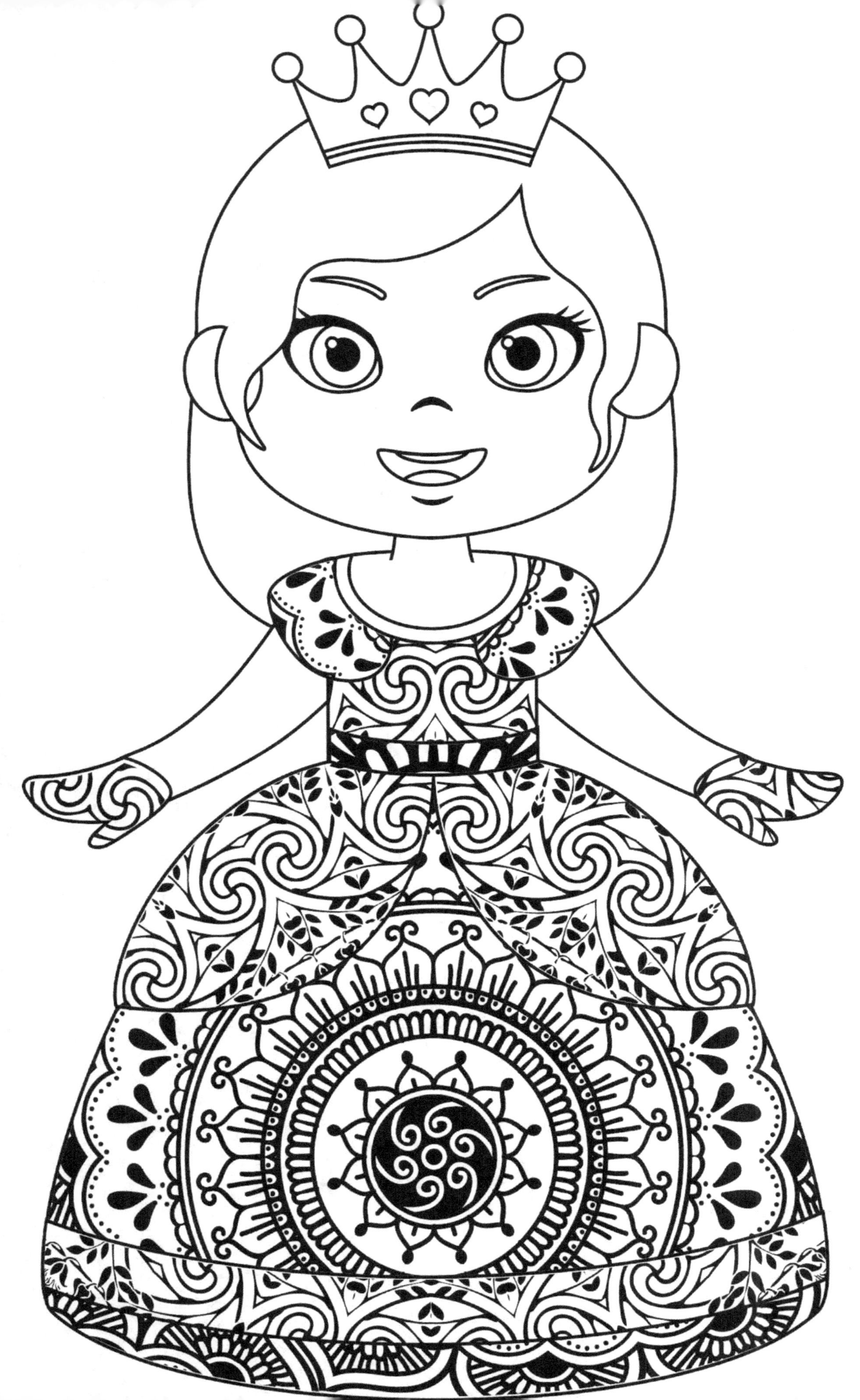

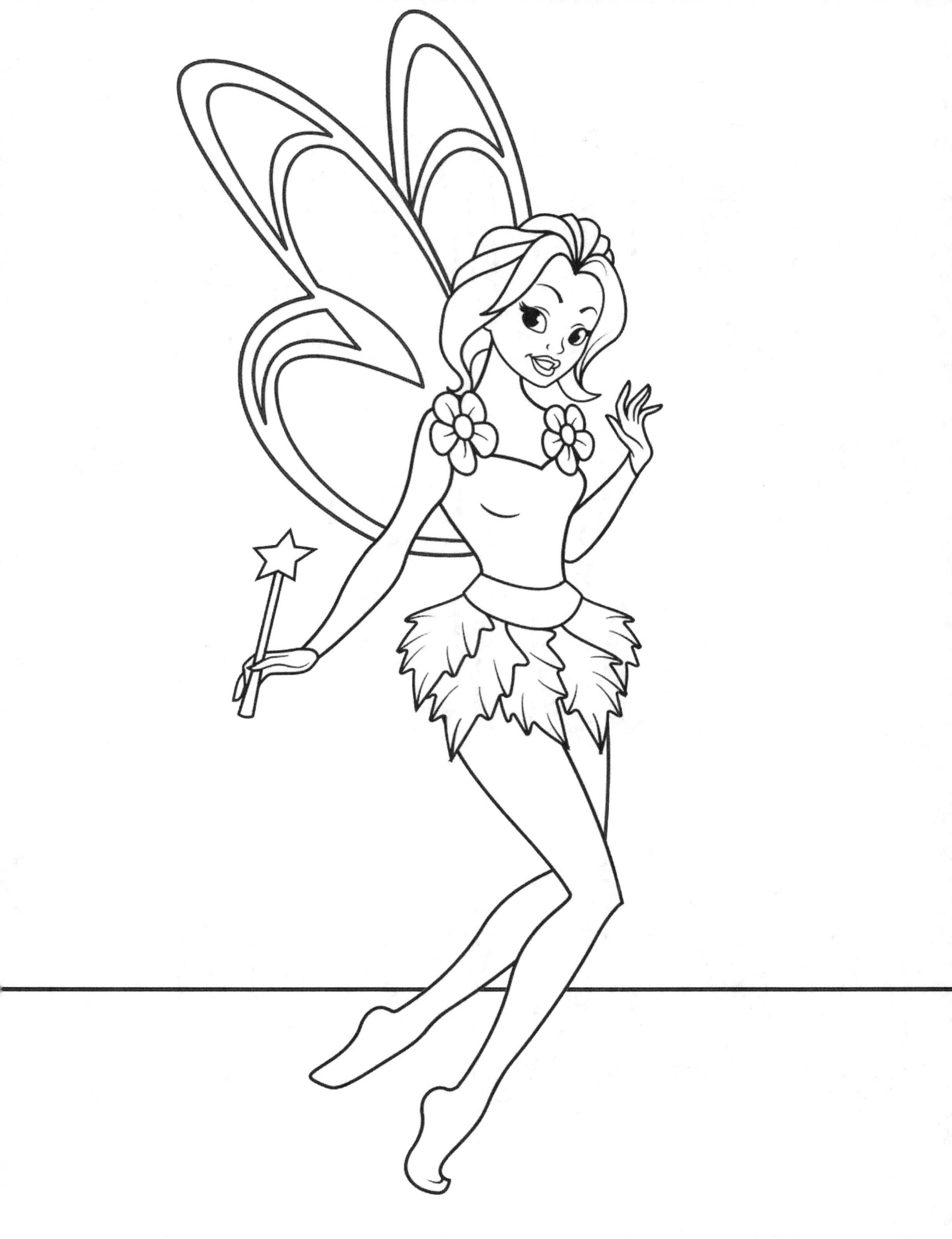

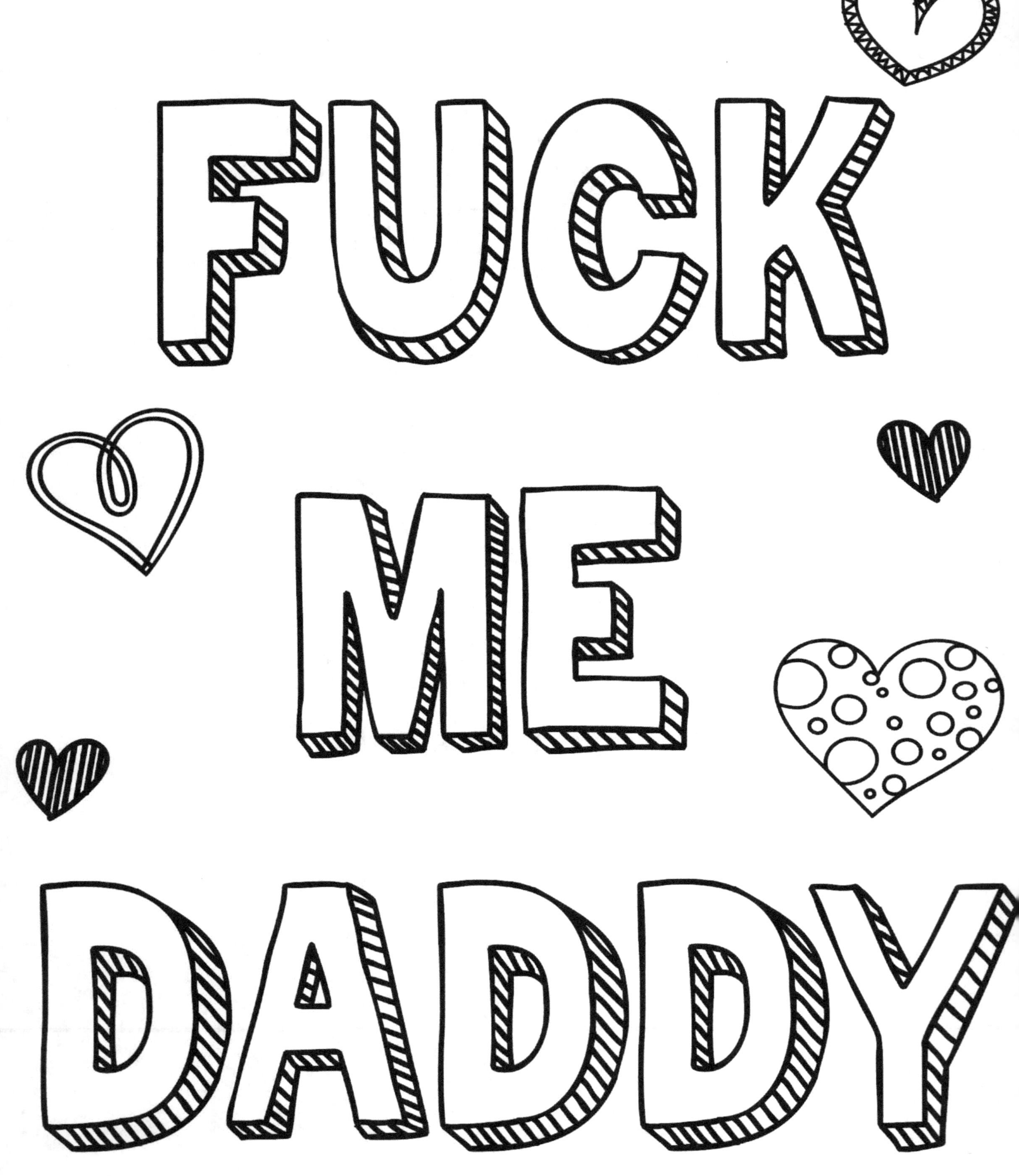

FUCK
ME
DADDY

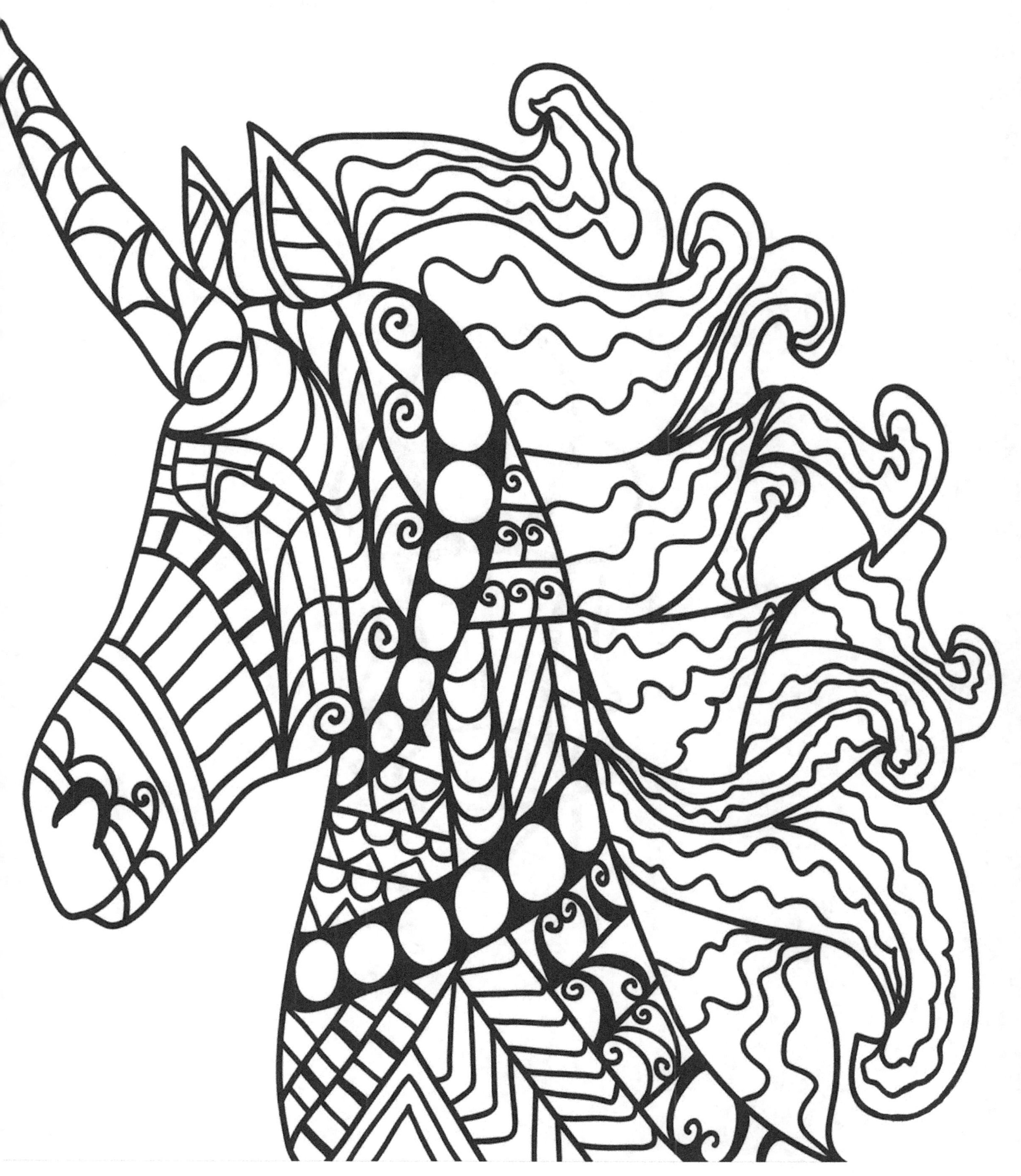

DRAW YOURSELF INTO THE LINGERIE FOR DADDY!

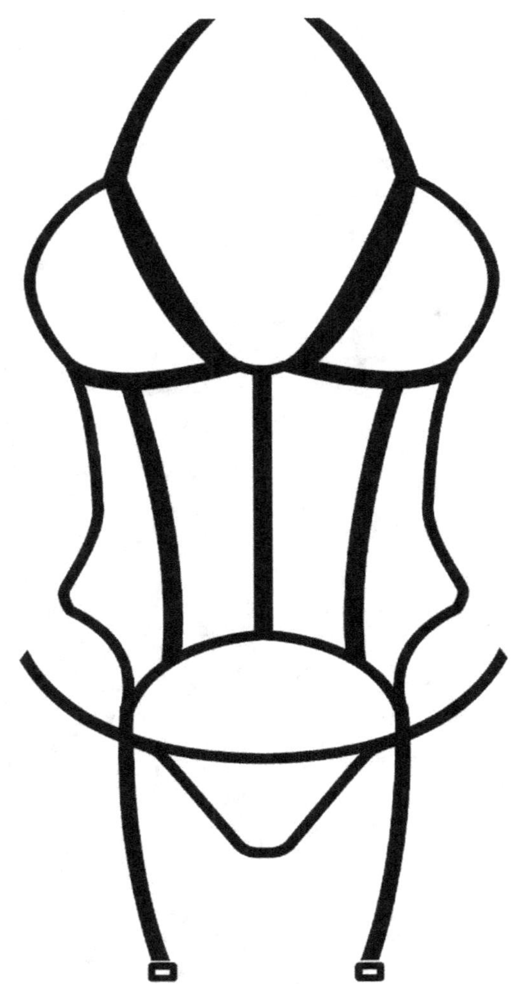

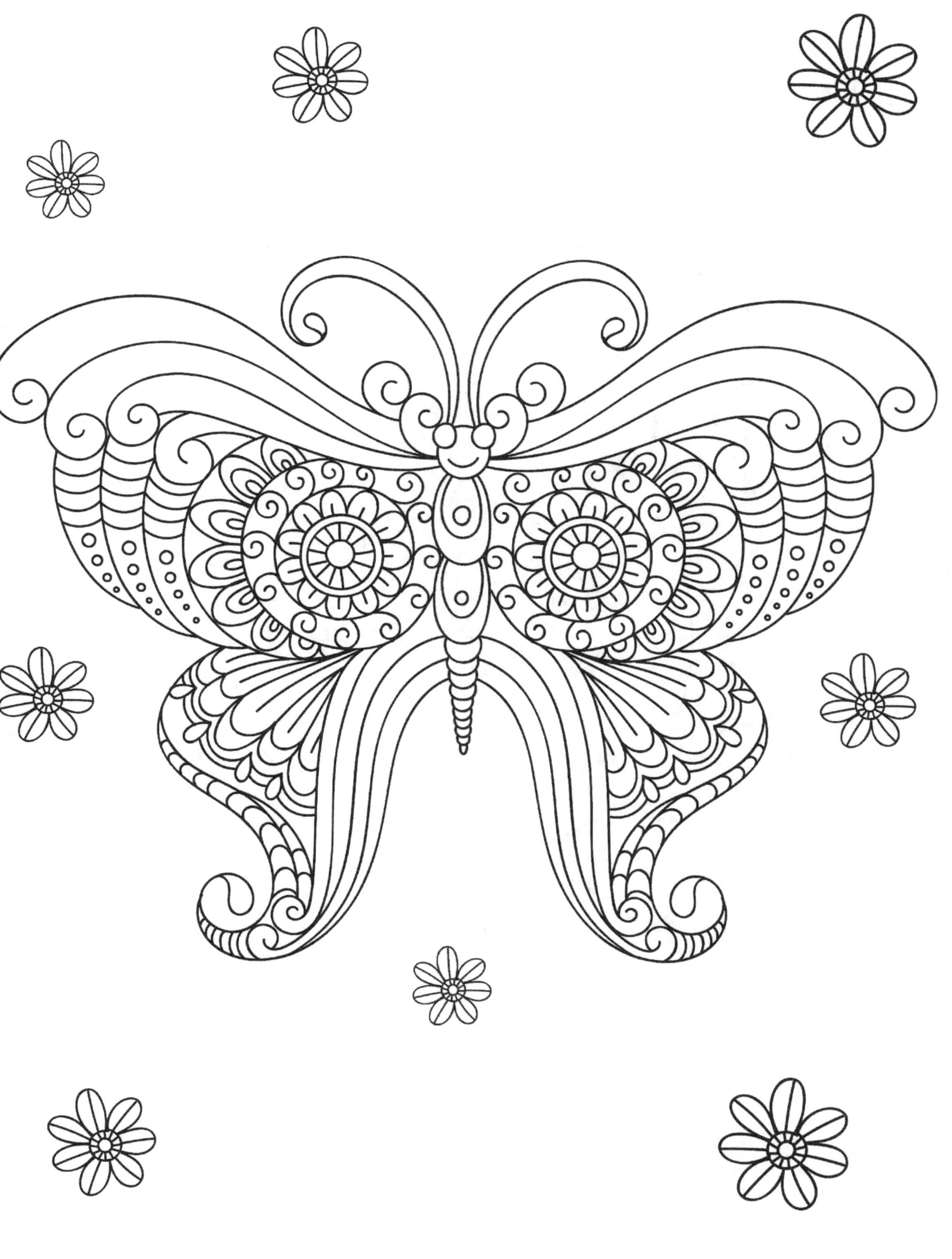

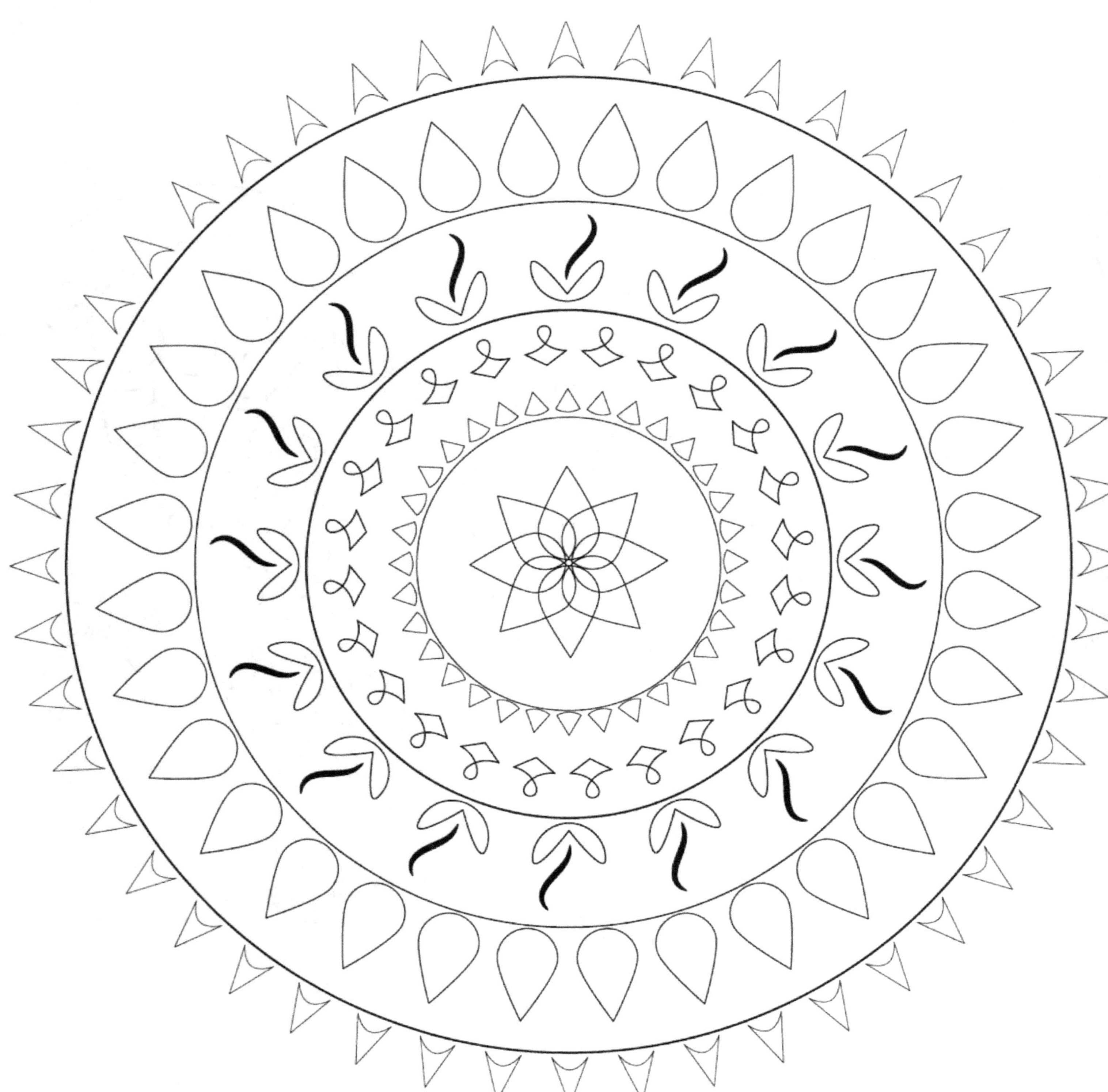

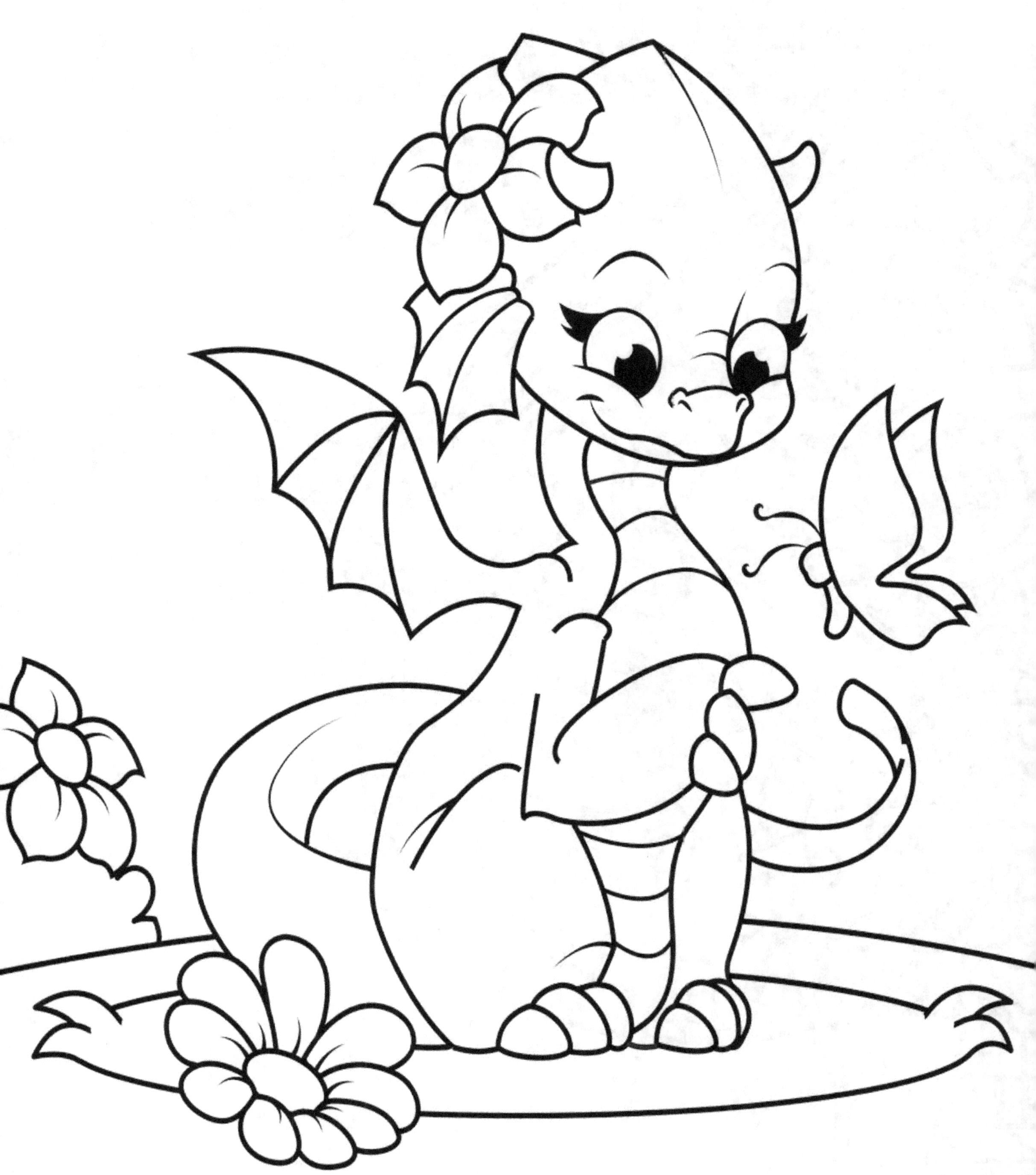

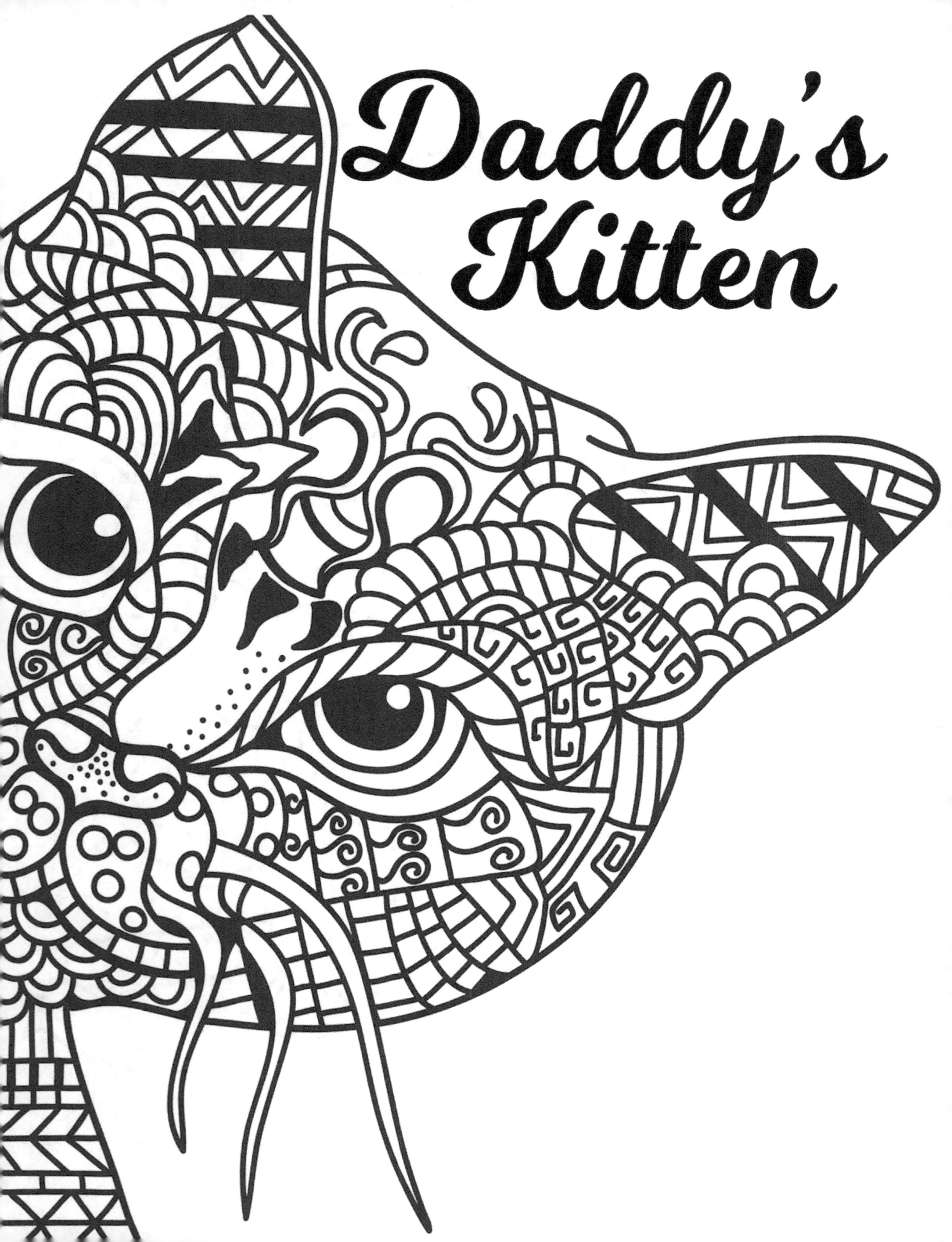
Daddy's
Kitten

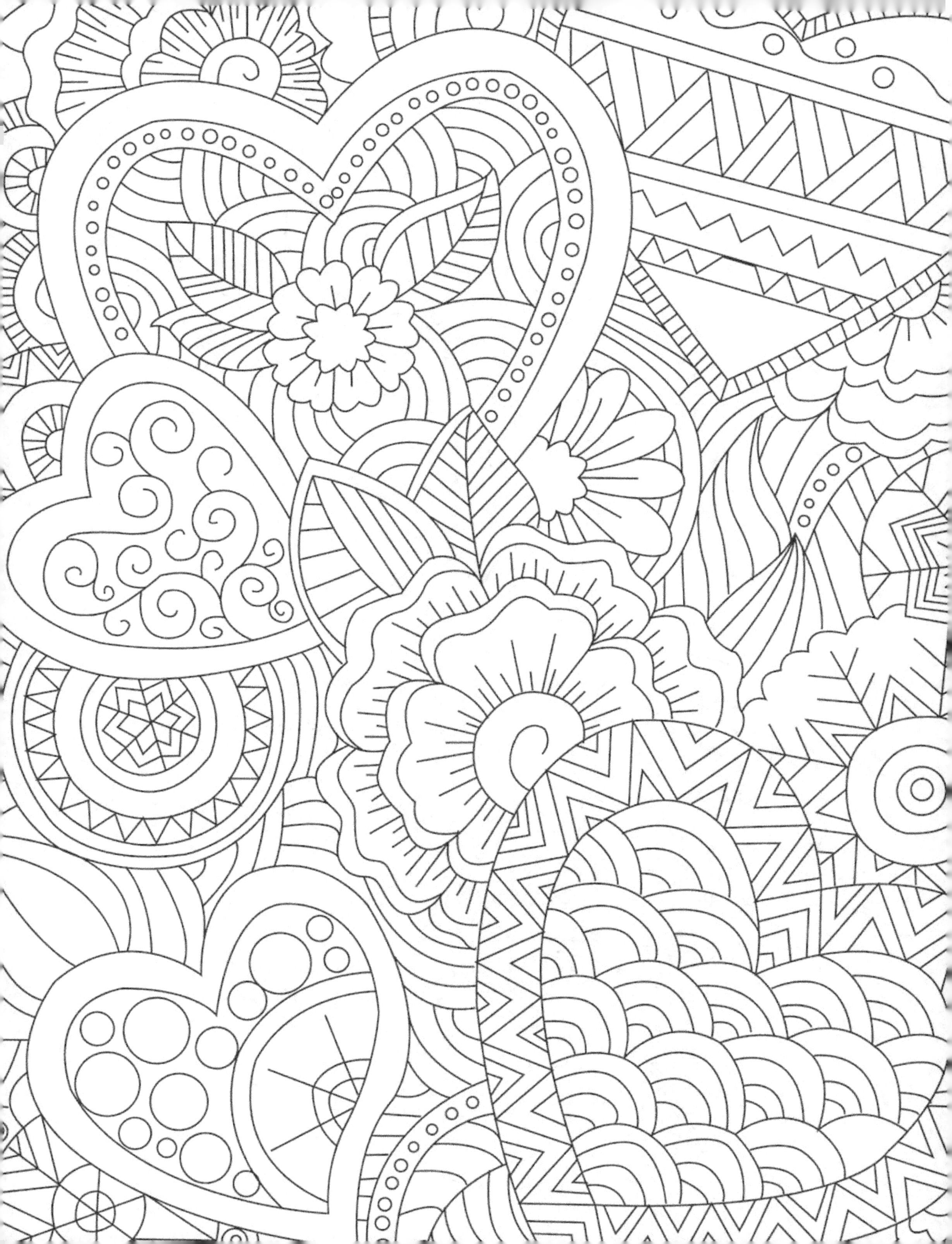

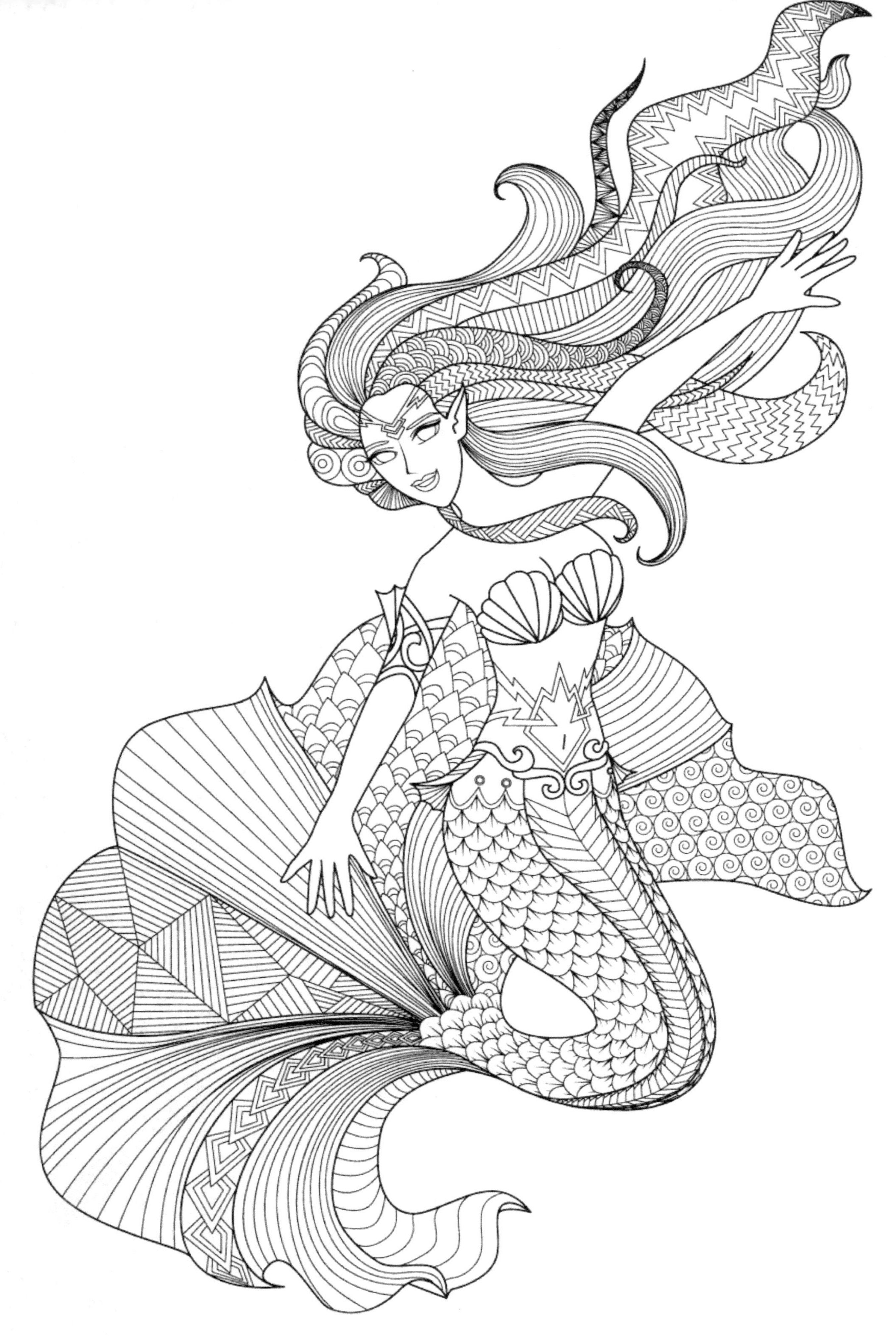

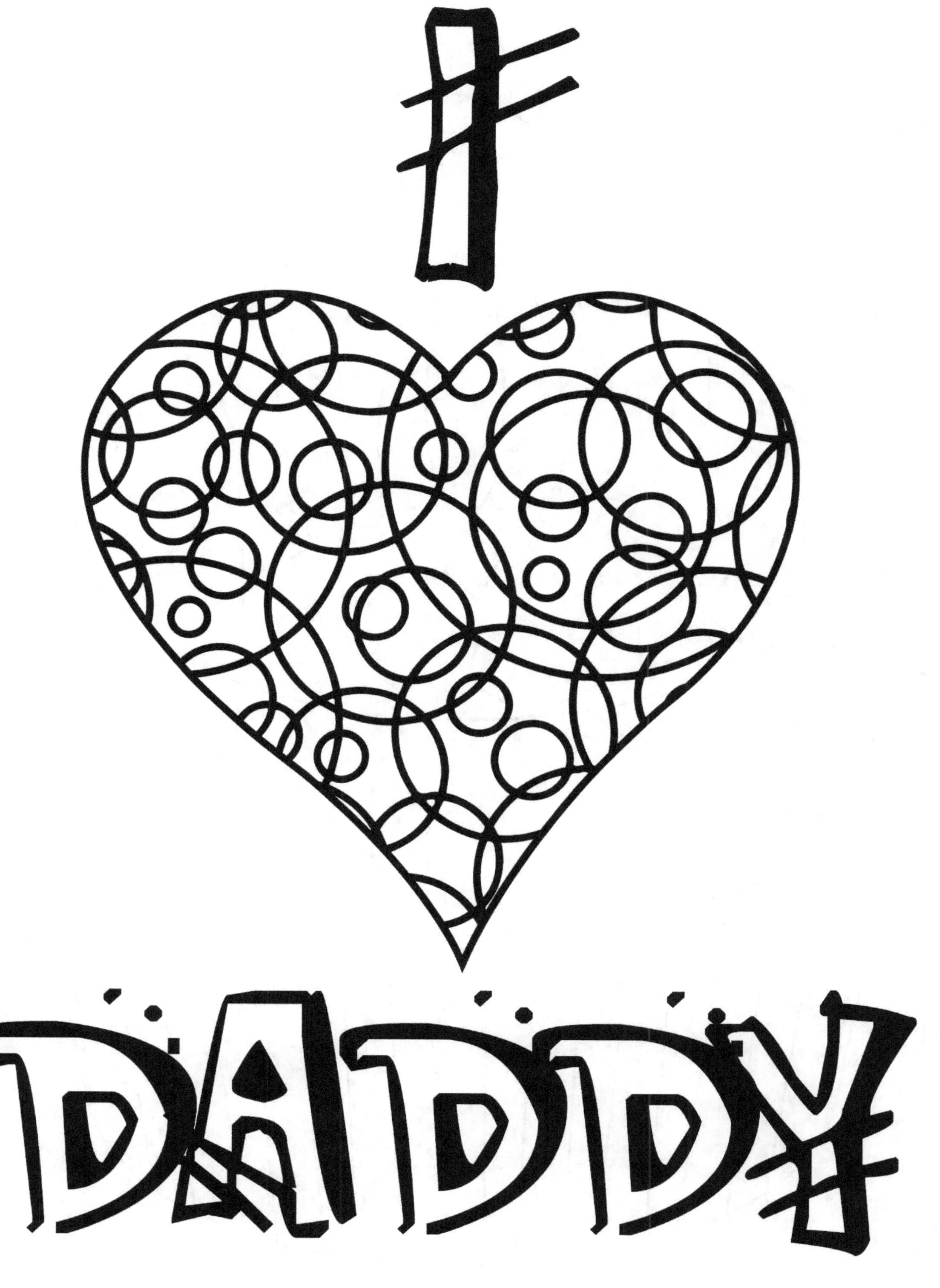
I
DADDY

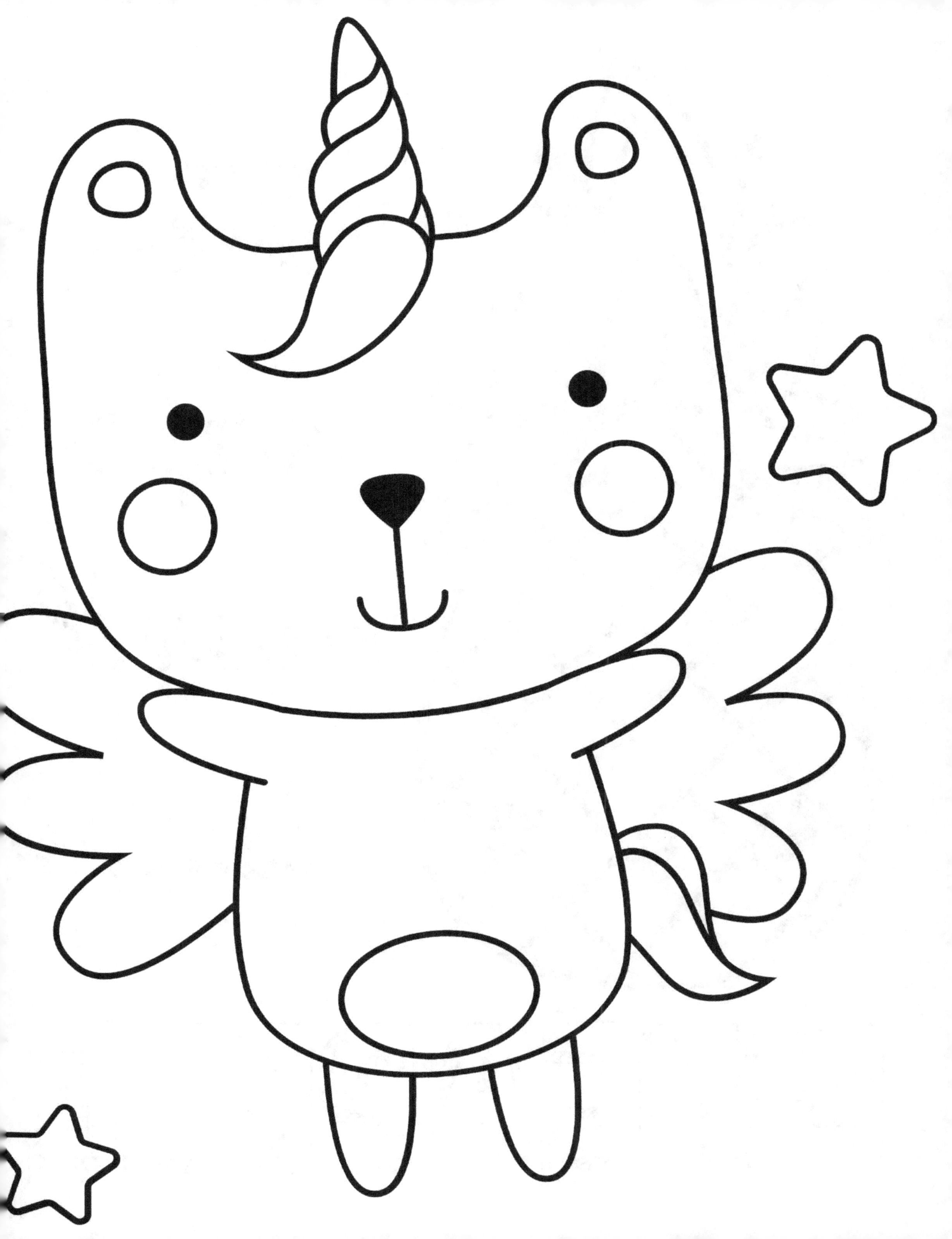

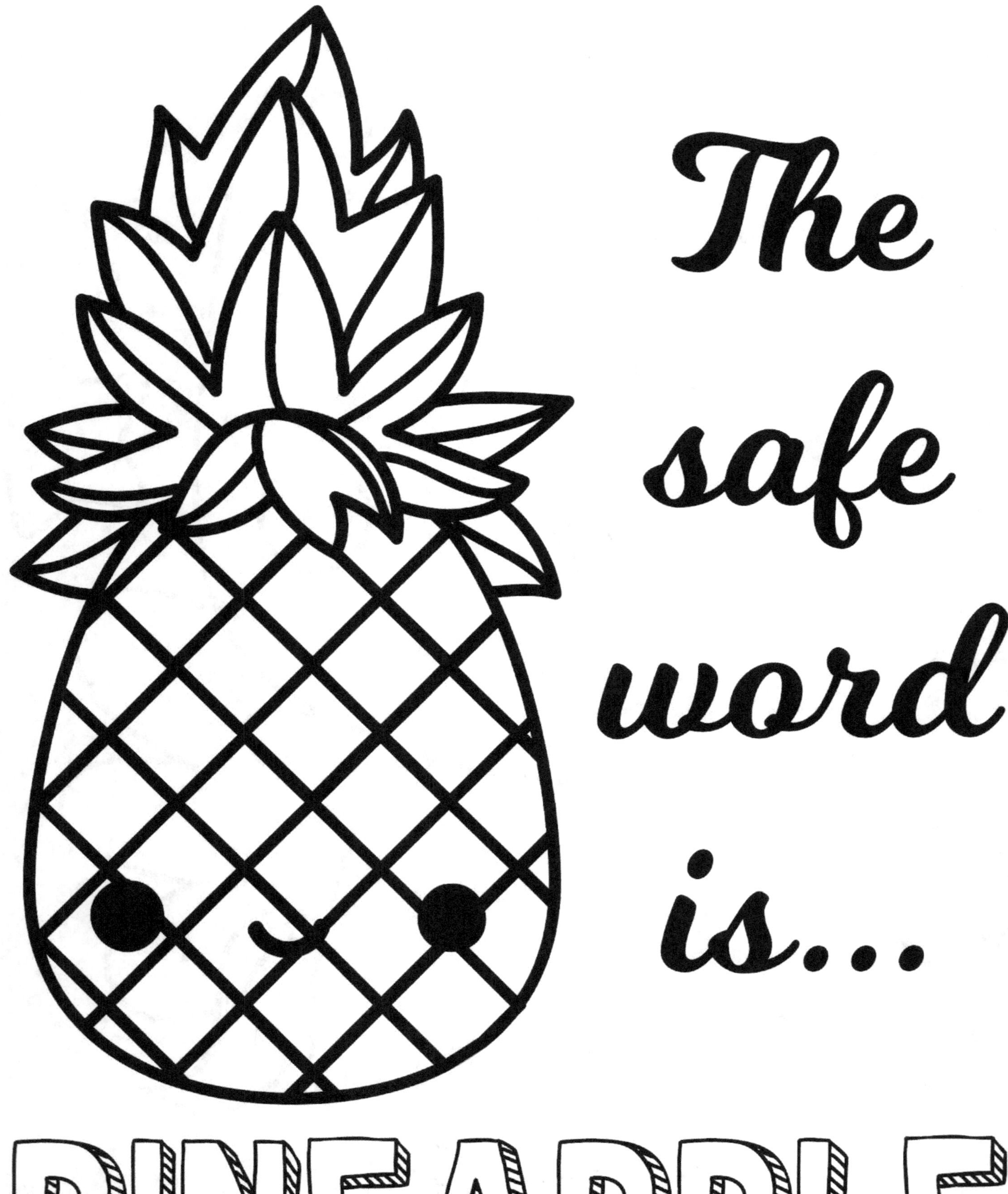
The
safe
word
is...
PINEAPPLE

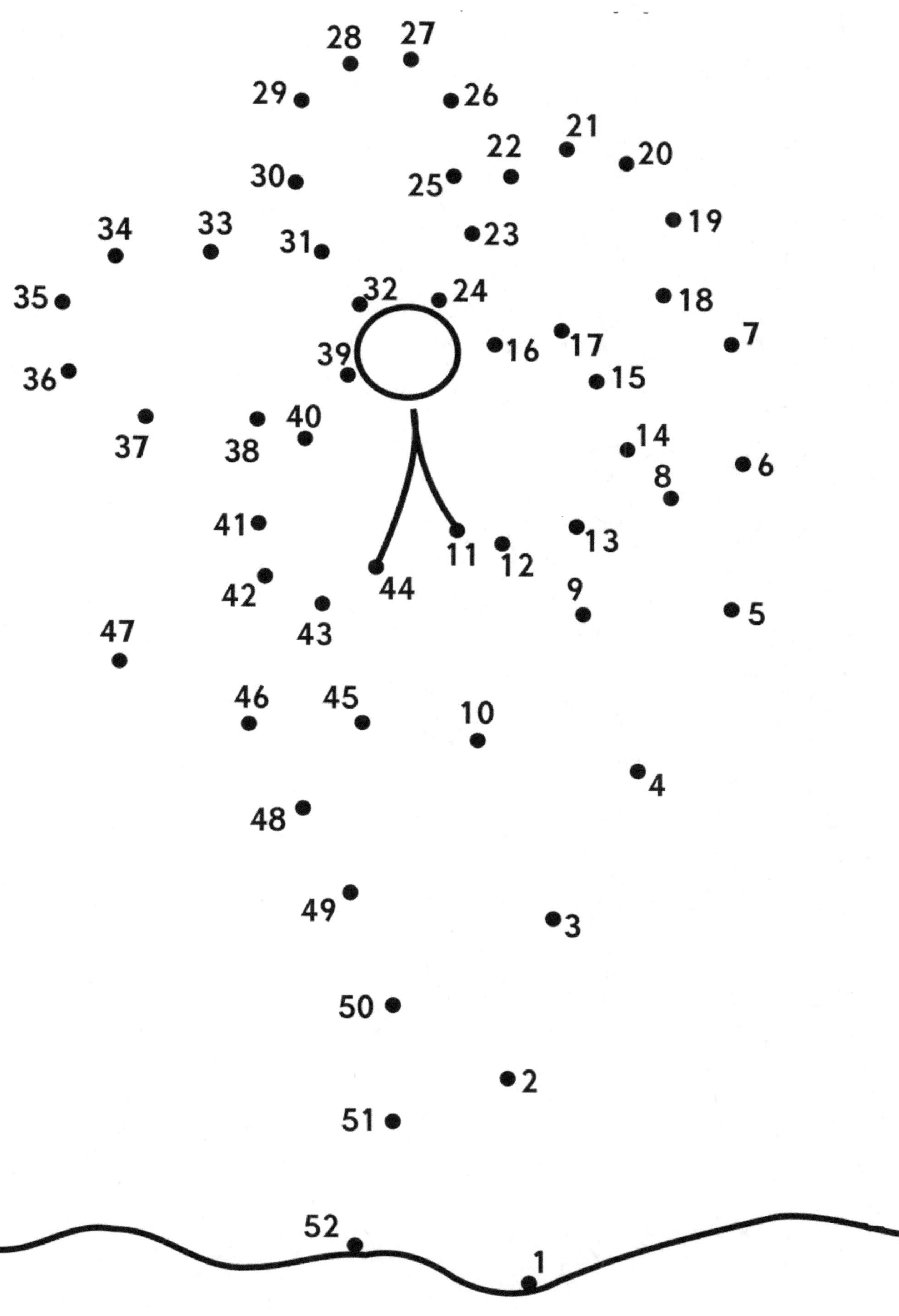

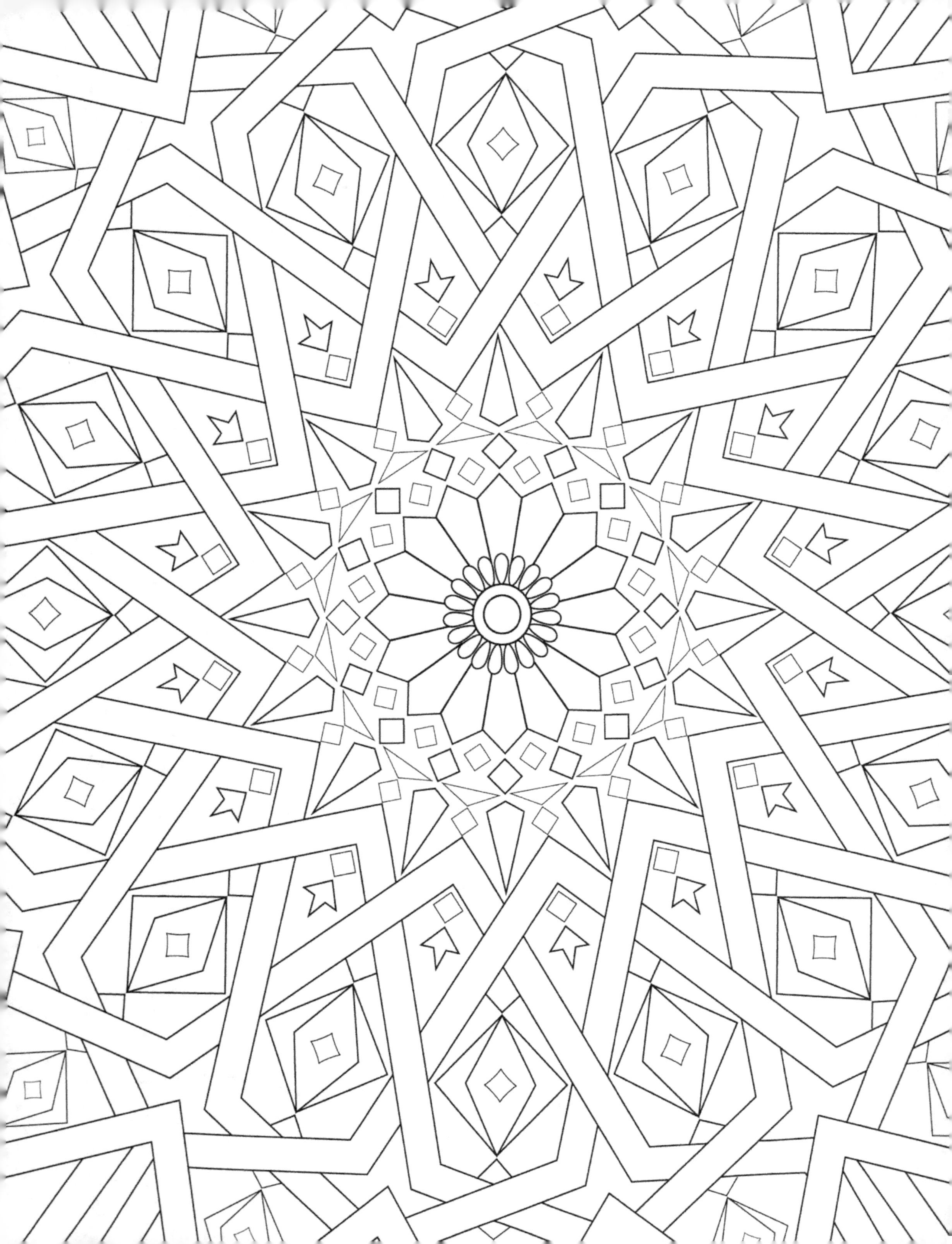

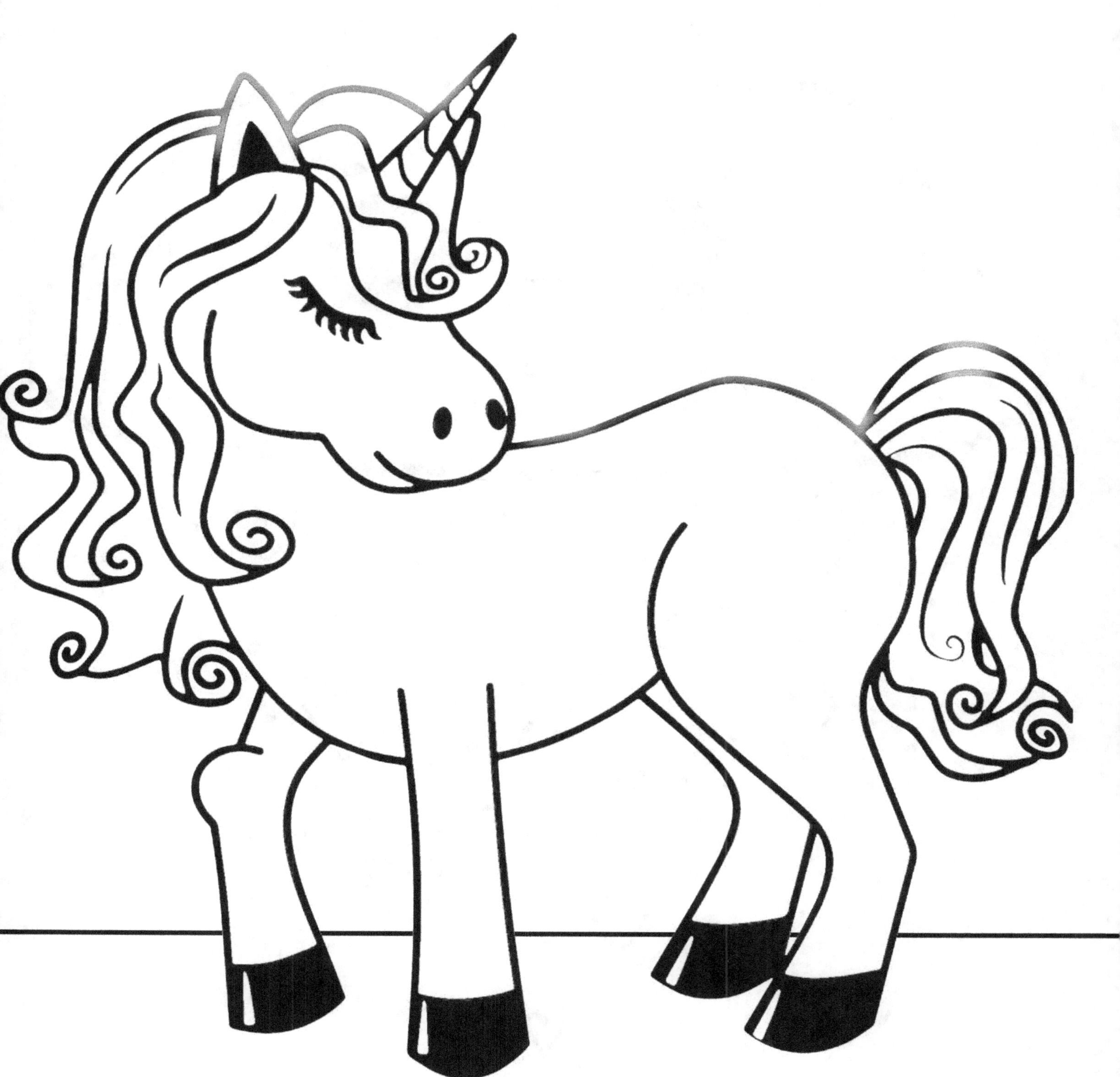

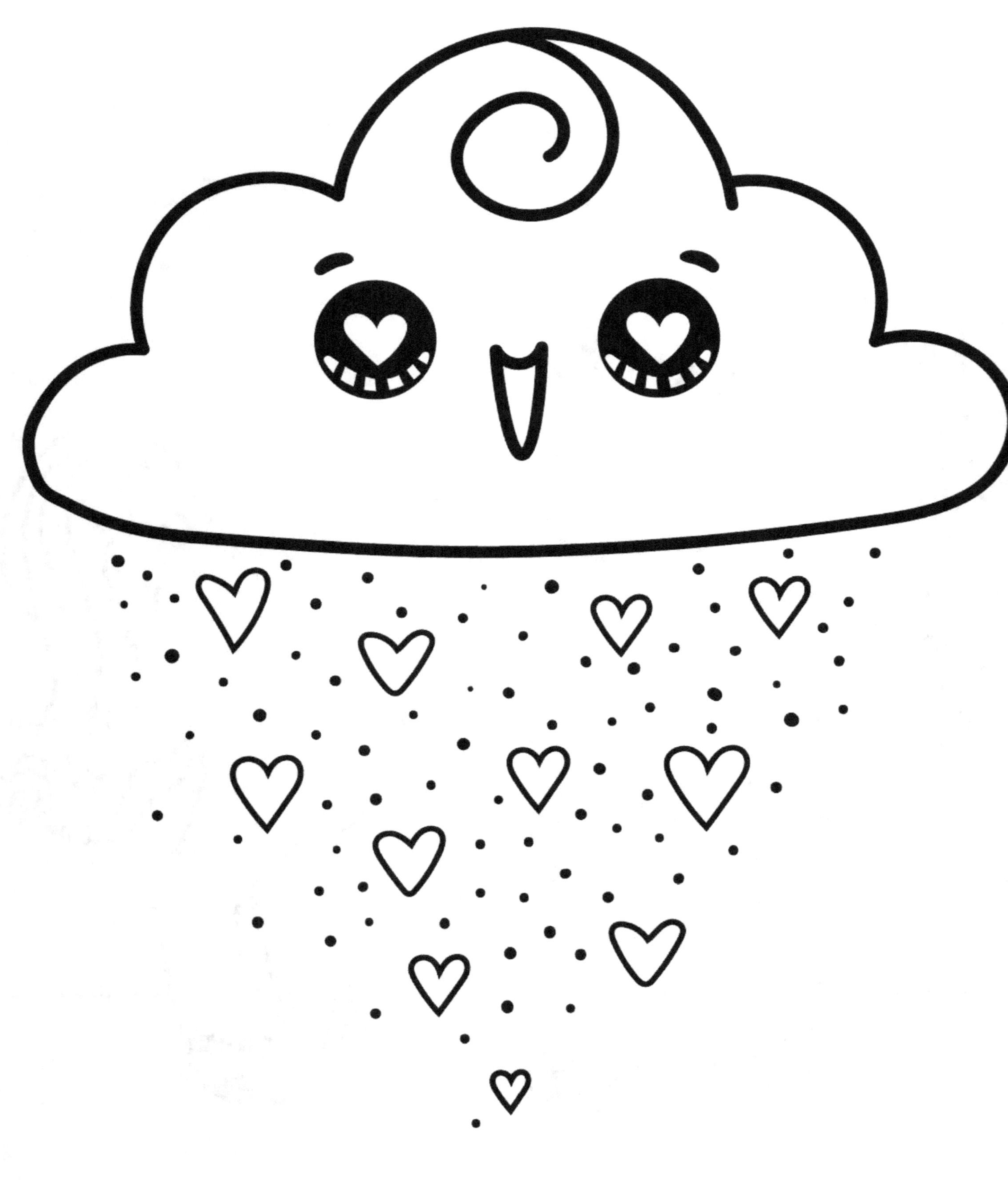

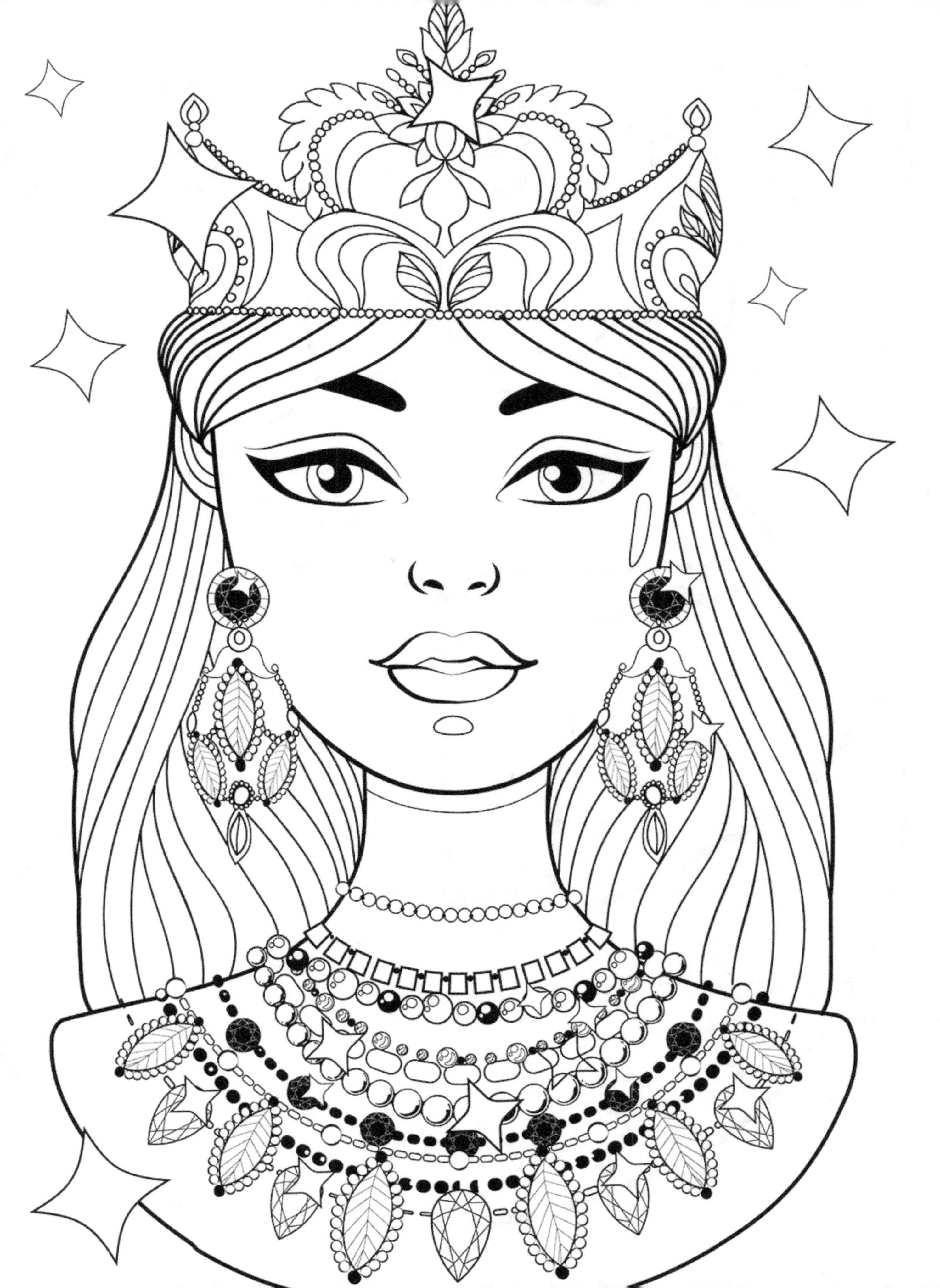

Little Fox

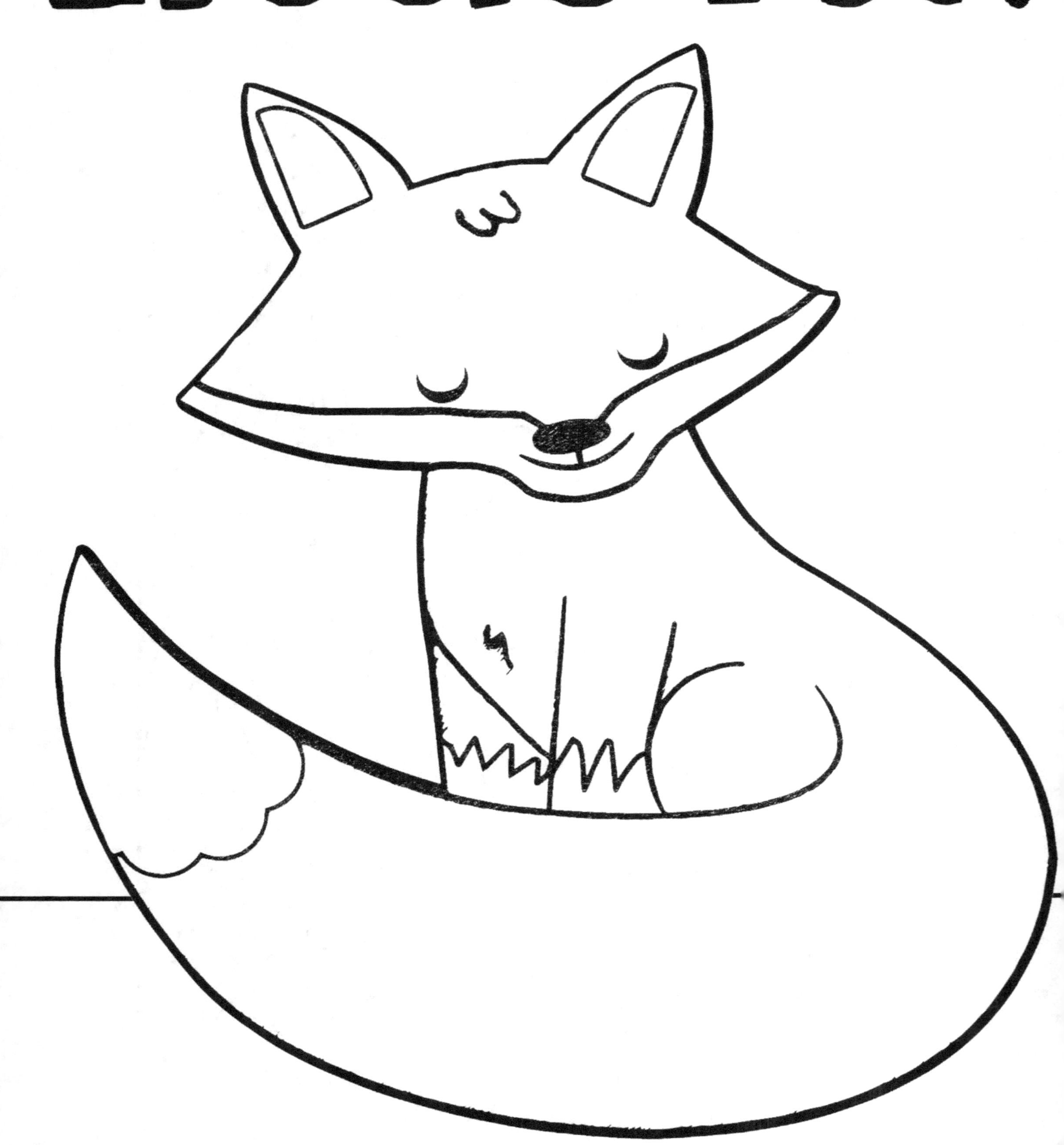

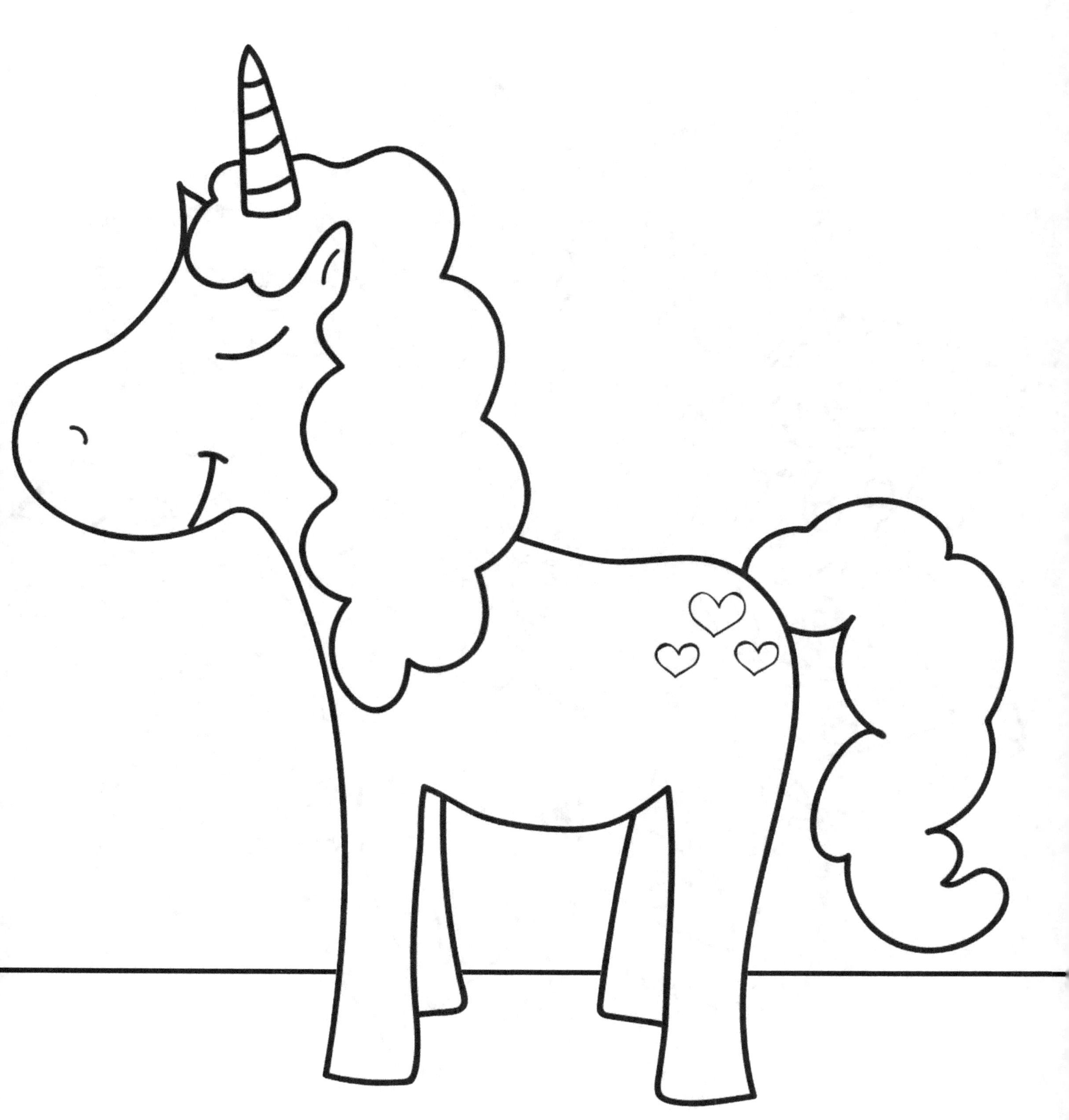

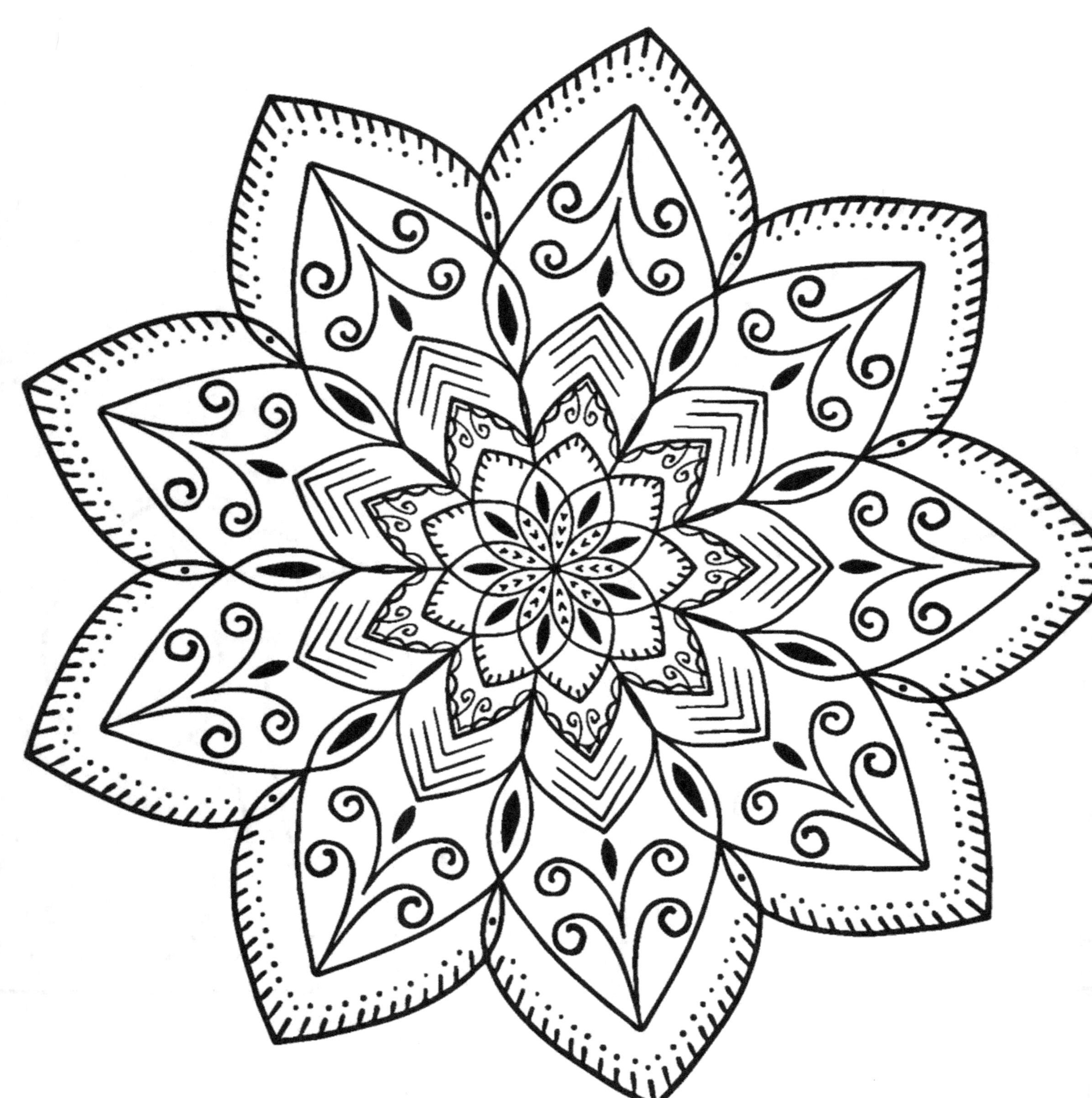

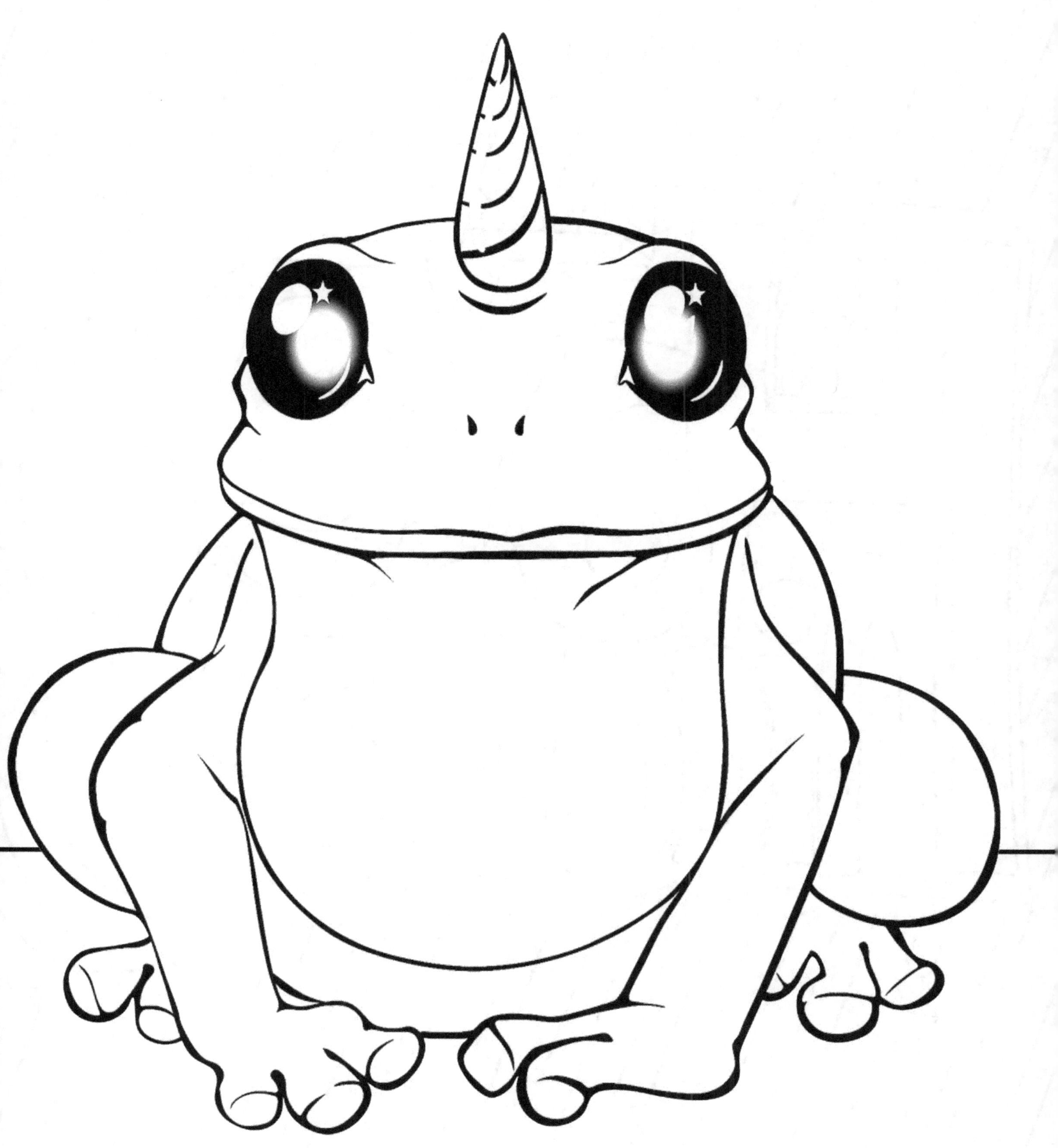

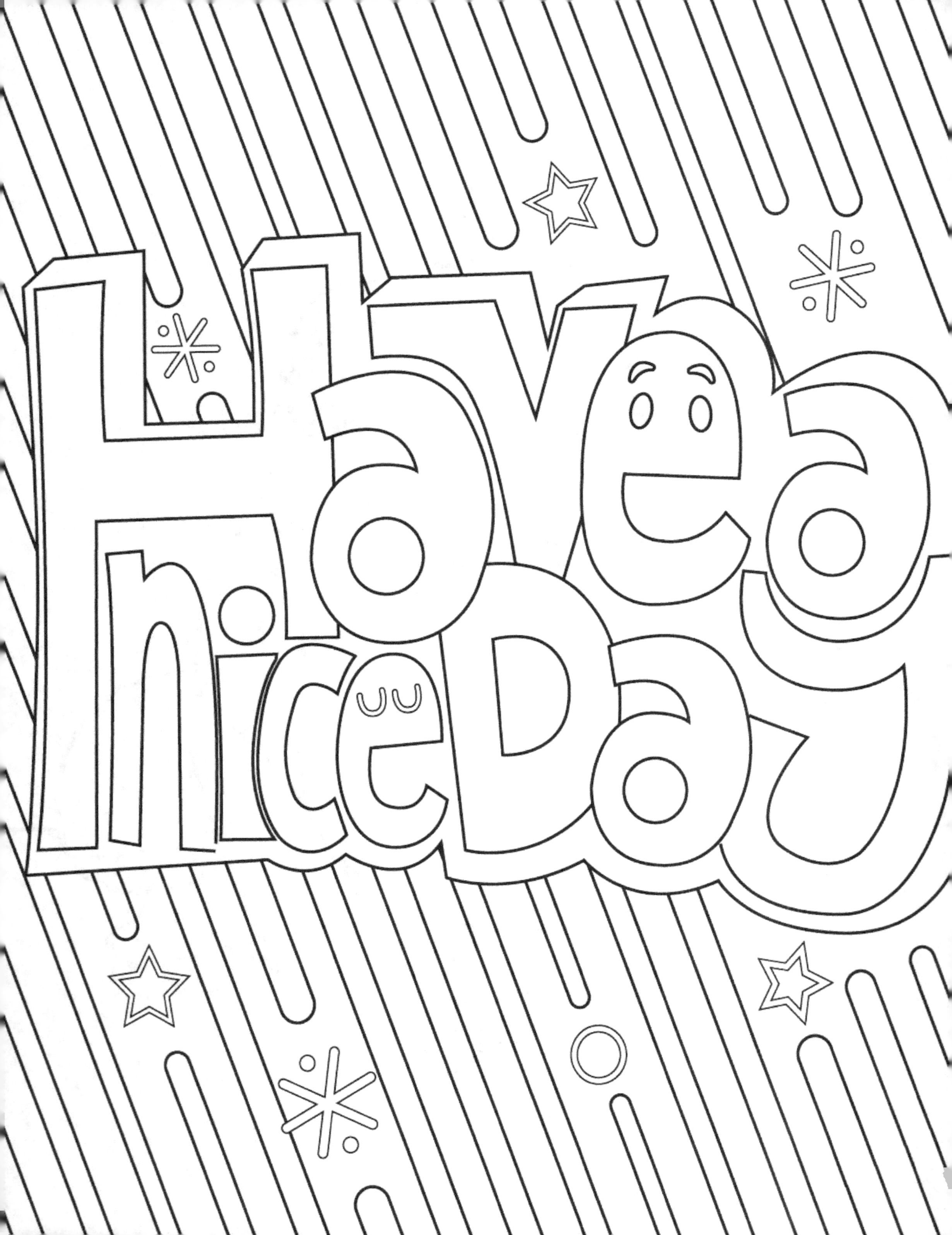

Have a nice Day

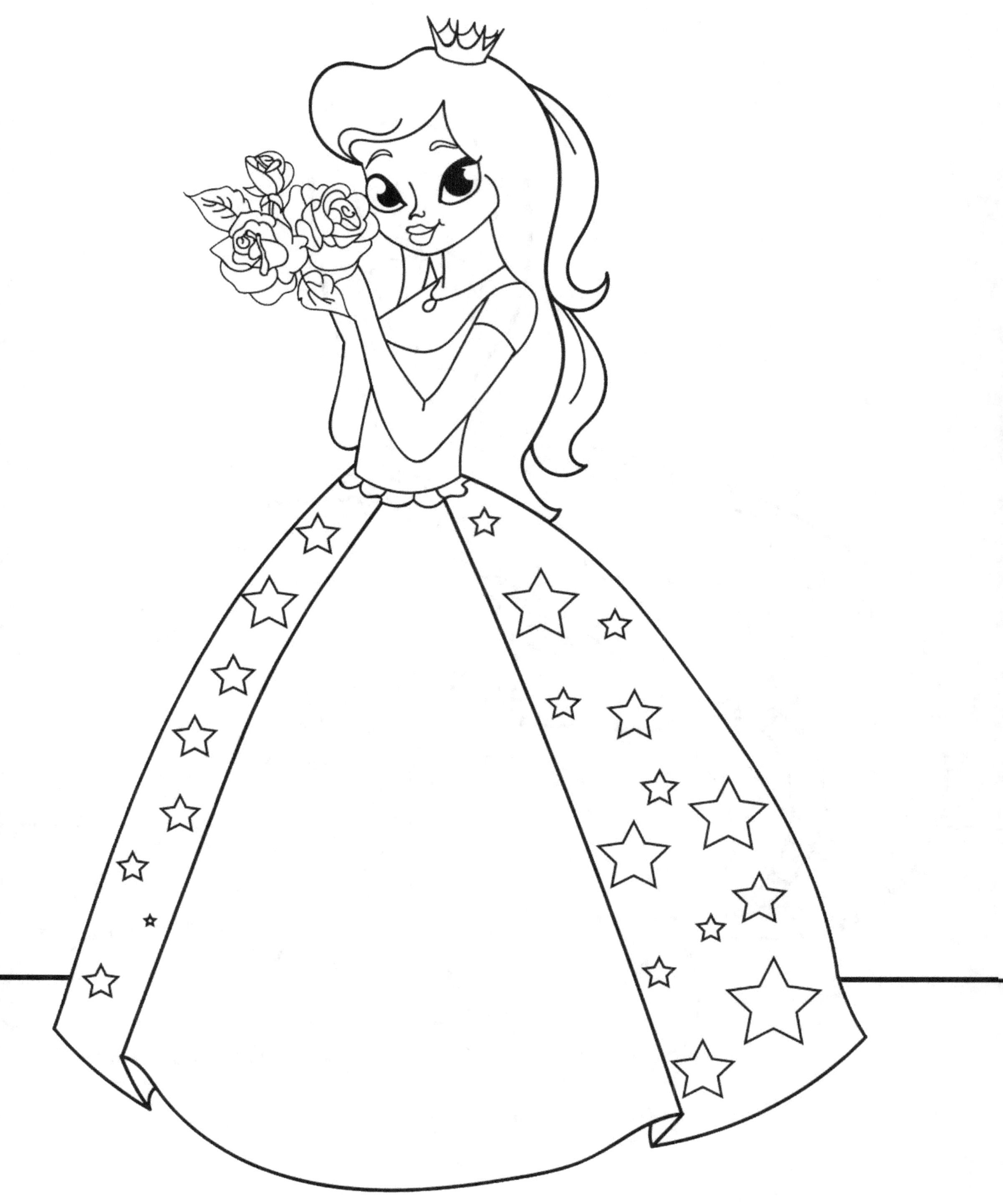

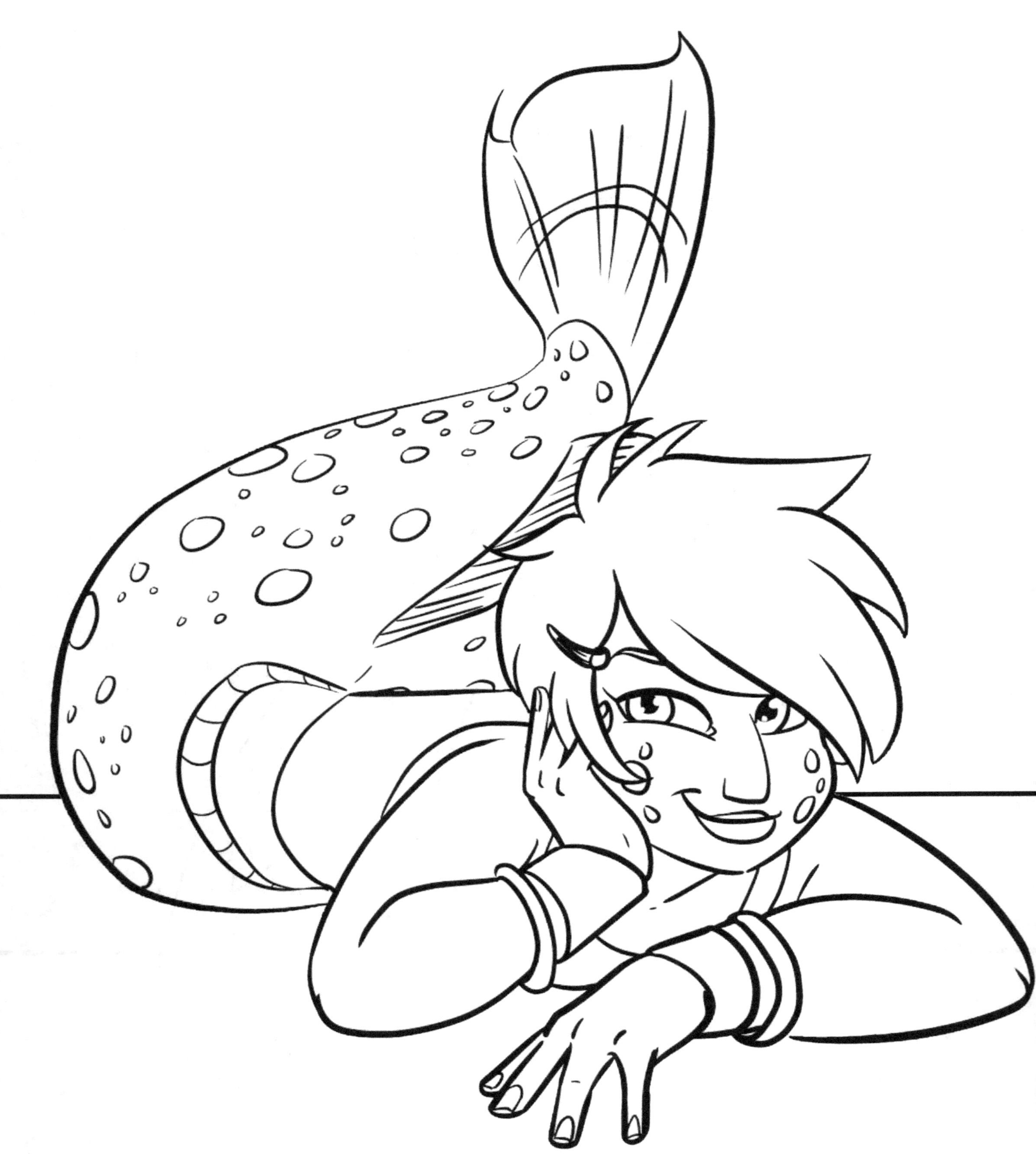

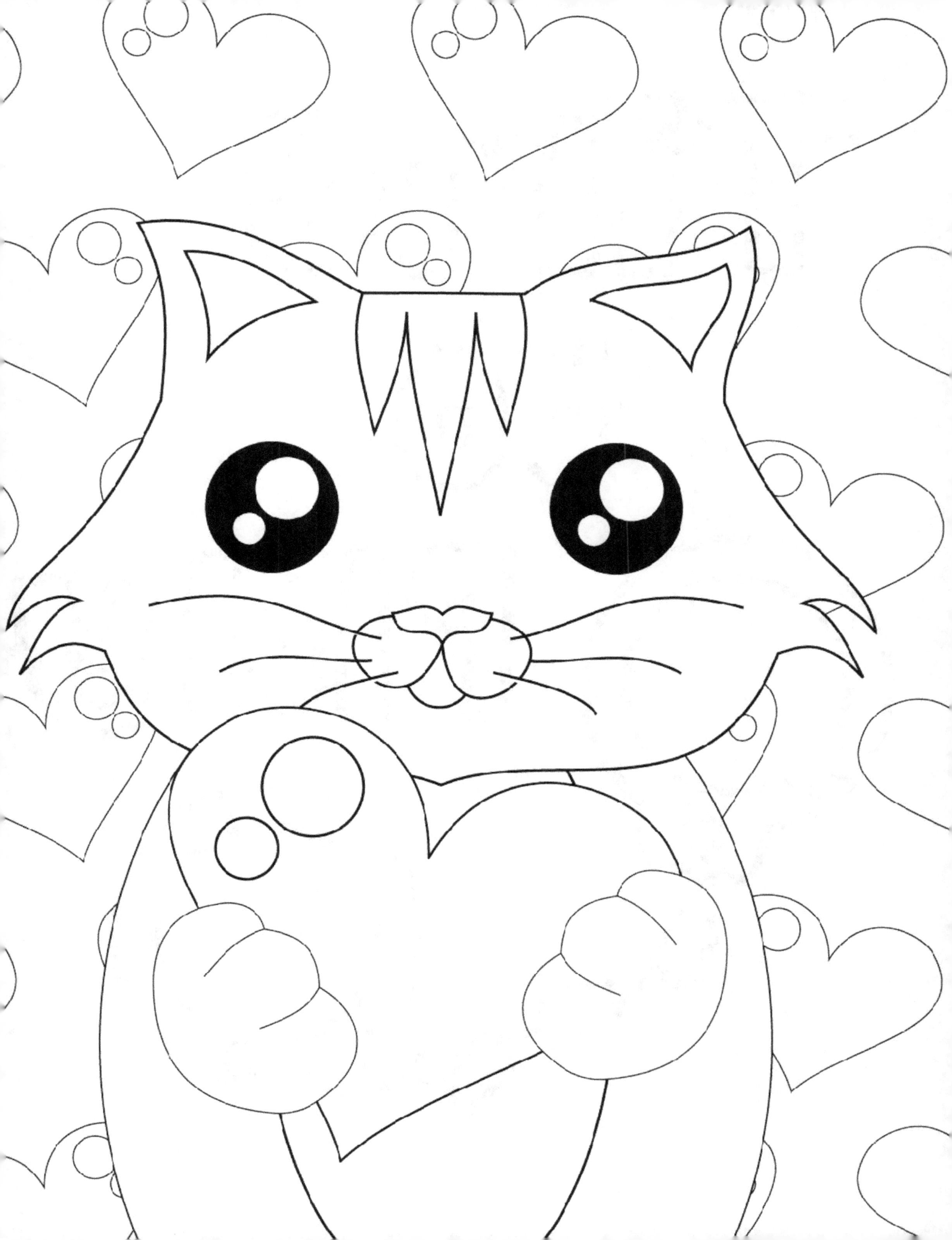

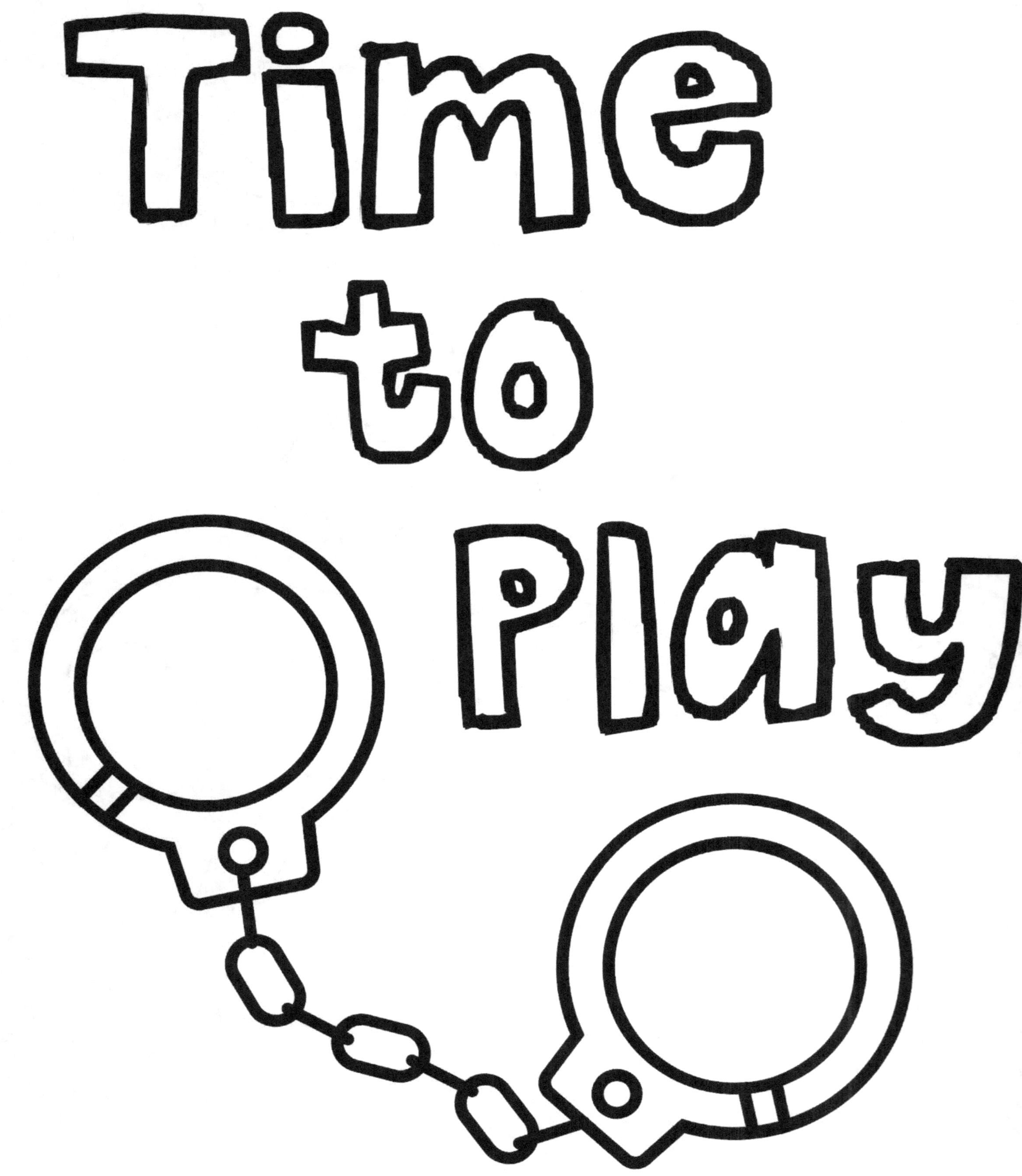

Time
to
Play

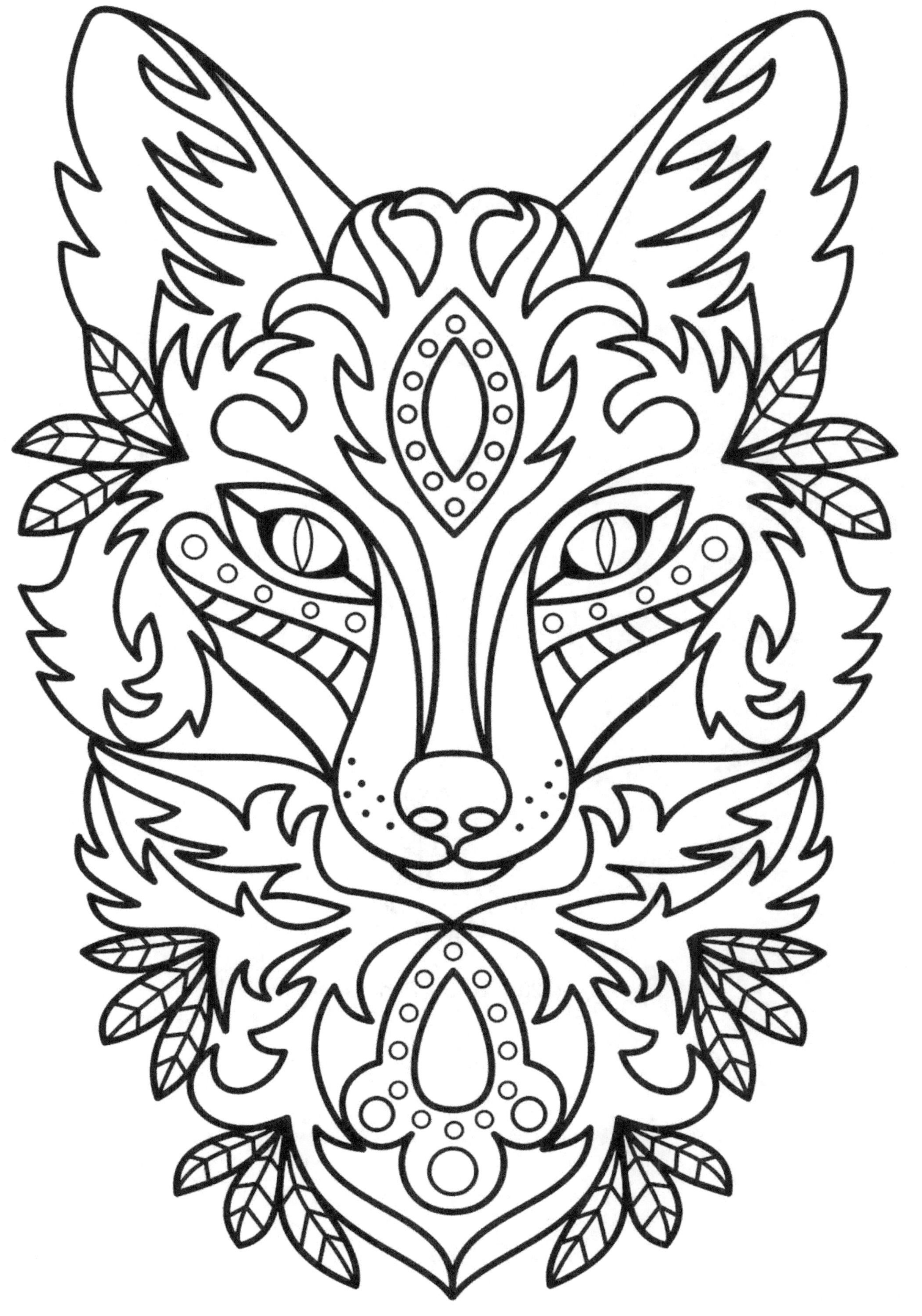

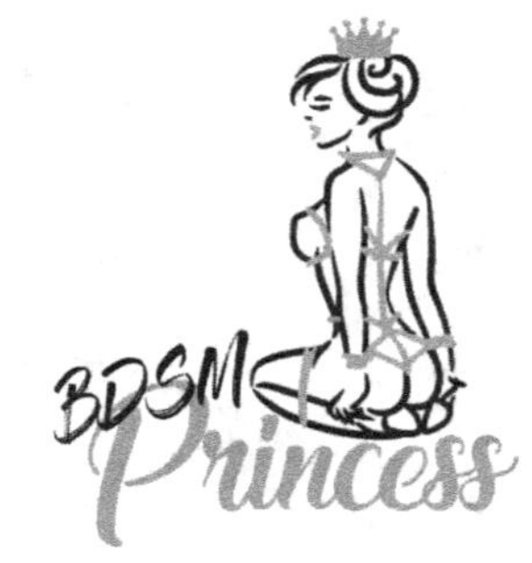

© 2019 BDSM Princess

Image Credits:
www.vecteezy.com
www.supercoloring.com

9 781693 897979